Table of Contents

1 Chapter 1: Cellular Defense Overview

Our bodies are constantly under siege. Invisible armies of viruses, bacteria, and other pathogens are perpetually trying to breach our defenses and establish themselves within us. Fortunately, we possess a sophisticated and multi-layered defense system to counter these threats. This complex interplay of cellular mechanisms and coordinated responses is what we call our immune system. Understanding the fundamentals of this system is crucial to appreciating how infectious diseases arise and, more importantly, how we can develop effective strategies to combat them.

The immune system operates on two primary fronts: innate immunity and adaptive immunity. Think of innate immunity as the first responders, the soldiers constantly patrolling the borders, ready to engage any invader immediately. It's a rapid, non-specific defense mechanism, meaning it doesn't target specific pathogens but rather recognizes general danger signals. These signals can be anything from the presence of foreign molecules like lipopolysaccharide (LPS) found in bacterial cell walls, to signs of cellular damage, such as the release of ATP or uric acid from injured cells. Cells of the innate immune system, such as macrophages, neutrophils, and natural killer (NK) cells, are equipped with pattern recognition receptors (PRRs) that bind to these danger signals, activating the immune response. This response can involve phagocytosis (engulfing and destroying pathogens), the release of inflammatory cytokines (chemical messengers that recruit other immune cells to the site of infection), and the activation of the complement system (a cascade of proteins that can directly kill pathogens or enhance phagocytosis). It's important to note, the innate response doesn't "remember" past encounters; it responds in the same way each time, providing immediate but short-lived protection. This initial response is absolutely critical in controlling the infection and buying time for the adaptive immune system to kick in.

Contrast that with adaptive immunity, which is the specialized forces that require reconnaissance and targeted training. This arm of the immune system is slower to respond, but it is highly specific and provides long-lasting protection. The key players in adaptive immunity are T and B lymphocytes. These cells have the remarkable ability to recognize specific antigens, which are molecules derived from pathogens or other foreign substances. T cells are further divided into helper T cells (Th cells) and cytotoxic T cells (Tc cells). Helper T cells are crucial for orchestrating the adaptive immune response. When a Th cell encounters an antigen presented by an antigen-presenting cell (APC), such as a dendritic cell, it becomes activated and releases cytokines that help activate other immune cells, including B cells and cytotoxic T cells. Cytotoxic T cells, on the other hand, are responsible for directly killing infected cells. They recognize antigens presented on the surface of infected cells and release cytotoxic molecules that induce apoptosis, or programmed cell death, in the target cell. It's a highly targeted attack, eliminating infected cells before the pathogen can replicate and spread. B lymphocytes are responsible for producing antibodies, also known as immunoglobulins. Antibodies are proteins that bind specifically to antigens, marking them for destruction or neutralization. There are different classes of antibodies (IgG, IgM, IgA, IgE, IgD), each with distinct functions and locations in the body. Some antibodies neutralize pathogens by preventing them from infecting cells. Others act as opsonins, enhancing phagocytosis by making it easier for phagocytes to engulf pathogens. Still others activate the complement system, leading to pathogen lysis. The beauty of adaptive immunity lies in its ability to generate immunological memory. After an initial encounter with an antigen, some T and B cells differentiate into memory cells. These memory cells are long-lived and can rapidly respond to subsequent encounters with the same antigen, providing long-lasting protection against infection. This is the basis for vaccination, where we introduce weakened or inactive pathogens into the body to generate immunological memory without causing disease.

Moreover, it's essential to recognize the intricate interplay between innate and adaptive immunity. The innate immune system not only provides immediate protection but also plays a crucial role in activating the adaptive immune response. For example, dendritic cells, which are part of the innate immune system, capture antigens at the site of infection and migrate to lymph nodes, where they present these antigens to T cells, initiating the adaptive immune response. Cytokines released by innate immune cells also influence the type of adaptive immune response that is generated. Furthermore, antibodies produced by B cells can enhance the activity of innate immune cells, such as macrophages and NK cells. This intricate cross-talk ensures a coordinated and effective immune response.

In essence, understanding this fundamental overview of cellular defense, encompassing both the immediate, broad-spectrum actions of innate immunity and the targeted, long-lasting capabilities of adaptive immunity, is vital. Without these defenses, our bodies would be constantly overwhelmed by the multitude of pathogens we encounter daily. The following chapters will delve into the specific mechanisms by which pathogens attempt to evade these defenses and the strategies we can employ to strengthen our immune system and protect ourselves from infectious diseases.

The complexity of the immune system is a testament to the evolutionary arms race between hosts and pathogens. Over millions of years, pathogens have evolved sophisticated strategies to evade our defenses, while our immune system has evolved equally sophisticated mechanisms to counter these threats.

Knowing the foundation of these processes is the initial step to unlocking the secrets of cellular orchestration against emerging infectious disease agents. It equips us with the necessary understanding to appreciate the challenges and opportunities in developing effective strategies to combat these threats.

1.1 Innate Immunity Basics

Innate immunity stands as the body's rapid-response force, an evolutionarily ancient system designed to immediately recognize and neutralize threats. Unlike its adaptive counterpart, innate immunity lacks immunological memory and provides a broad, non-specific defense against a wide range of pathogens. Think of it as the first line of defense – the castle walls, moats, and vigilant guards – working tirelessly to prevent invaders from gaining a foothold. Its effectiveness hinges on rapid recognition and activation of various cellular and molecular components.

This initial recognition is largely mediated by pattern recognition receptors (PRRs). These receptors, expressed on various immune cells like macrophages, dendritic cells, and neutrophils, recognize conserved molecular patterns known as pathogen-associated molecular patterns (PAMPs). PAMPs are unique to microbes and are essential for their survival, making them reliable targets for the immune system. Examples include lipopolysaccharide (LPS) found in Gram-negative bacteria, peptidoglycan in Gram-positive bacteria, and viral nucleic acids like double-stranded RNA. PRRs also recognize damage-associated molecular patterns (DAMPs), released from damaged or stressed host cells, alerting the immune system to tissue injury. This dual recognition system ensures that the innate immune system can respond to both infectious agents and cellular damage. This is also where your body starts to create something to fight the invaders.

Once a PRR binds to a PAMP or DAMP, a cascade of intracellular signaling pathways is activated. These pathways lead to the production and release of inflammatory cytokines and chemokines. Cytokines are signaling molecules that orchestrate the immune response, promoting inflammation, recruiting immune cells to the site of infection, and activating other immune cells. Chemokines, on the other hand, act as chemoattractants, guiding immune cells to the infected tissue. The release of these mediators creates a local inflammatory environment, characterized by redness, swelling, heat, and pain, which is essential for clearing the infection. This allows the body to react to threats immediately.

Among the key cellular players in innate immunity are phagocytes: macrophages, neutrophils, and dendritic cells. Macrophages, residing in tissues throughout the body, are versatile cells that engulf and destroy pathogens through phagocytosis. They also act as antigen-presenting cells, bridging the innate and adaptive immune responses by presenting processed antigens to T cells. Neutrophils, the most abundant type of white blood cell, are rapidly recruited to the site of infection, where they phagocytose and kill bacteria and other pathogens. Dendritic cells, strategically located in tissues that are in contact with the external environment, capture antigens and migrate to lymph nodes, where they activate T cells, initiating the adaptive immune response. Each type of cell has a specific role, allowing the innate immune system to work on multiple aspects to get rid of invaders.

The complement system is another crucial component of innate immunity, comprising a cascade of plasma proteins that are activated upon recognition of pathogens. Complement activation leads to several outcomes, including opsonization, which enhances phagocytosis; direct lysis of pathogens; and recruitment of inflammatory cells. There are three pathways of complement activation: the classical pathway, triggered by antibody-antigen complexes; the alternative pathway, activated by direct binding of complement proteins to pathogen surfaces; and the lectin pathway, initiated by binding of mannose-binding lectin (MBL) to mannose residues on pathogens. Activation of any of these pathways converges on the formation of C3 convertase, which cleaves C3 into C3a and C3b, initiating the downstream effects of complement.

Natural killer (NK) cells are lymphocytes that play a critical role in eliminating virus-infected cells and tumor cells. Unlike T cells, NK cells do not require prior sensitization or antigen presentation to become activated. They recognize target cells through a balance of activating and inhibitory receptors. Activating receptors recognize stress-induced ligands on target cells, while inhibitory receptors recognize MHC class I molecules, which are expressed on healthy cells. If the activating signals outweigh the inhibitory signals, the NK cell is activated, releasing cytotoxic granules that kill the target cell. This mechanism ensures that NK cells selectively eliminate infected or cancerous cells without harming healthy cells.

Epithelial barriers, such as the skin and mucous membranes, form the first physical barrier against pathogen entry. These barriers are tightly sealed by tight junctions, preventing pathogens from penetrating into the underlying tissues. In addition, epithelial surfaces secrete antimicrobial substances, such as defensins and cathelicidins, which directly kill bacteria and viruses. The mucociliary escalator in the respiratory tract traps pathogens in mucus and sweeps them away from the lungs. The acidic environment of the stomach also kills many ingested pathogens. These physical and chemical barriers provide a constant defense against infection, preventing pathogens from even gaining access to the body.

1.2 Adaptive Response Primer

The adaptive immune response, unlike its innate counterpart, is not immediate. It requires a period of sensitization, where immune cells encounter and recognize specific antigens associated with the invading pathogen. This recognition process is the cornerstone of adaptive immunity, allowing for a tailored and highly effective response. Unlike the broad, non-specific mechanisms of innate immunity, the adaptive response possesses exquisite specificity, capable of distinguishing between closely related pathogens or even different strains of the same pathogen. This level of precision is achieved through the action of lymphocytes, specifically T cells and B cells, each with unique antigen receptors.

The process begins with antigen presentation. Innate immune cells, such as dendritic cells, engulf pathogens and process their proteins into smaller peptide fragments. These peptide fragments, or antigens, are then displayed on the surface of the dendritic cell bound to Major Histocompatibility Complex (MHC) molecules. MHC molecules come in two main classes: MHC class I, which presents antigens derived from intracellular pathogens (e.g., viruses) to cytotoxic T cells (also known as CD8+ T cells), and MHC class II, which presents antigens derived from extracellular pathogens (e.g., bacteria) to helper T cells (also known as CD4+ T cells). The presentation of antigen by dendritic cells is not merely a passive display; it's a critical step in activating the adaptive immune response. These dendritic cells then migrate to lymph nodes, the central meeting places for immune cells, where they interact with T cells.

T cell activation is a highly regulated process that requires two signals. The first signal is the interaction between the T cell receptor (TCR) on the T cell and the antigen-MHC complex on the dendritic cell. This interaction is highly specific; each TCR is designed to recognize a unique antigen. However, this first signal alone is not sufficient to activate the T cell. A second signal, known as a co-stimulatory signal, is also required. This signal is typically provided by the interaction of co-stimulatory molecules on the dendritic cell with co-stimulatory receptors on the T cell. Without the co-stimulatory signal, the T cell may become anergic, meaning it becomes unresponsive to future antigen stimulation. Once a T cell is fully activated, it proliferates and differentiates into effector T cells, which are specialized to carry out specific immune functions. CD8+ T cells differentiate into cytotoxic T lymphocytes (CTLs), which can kill infected cells. CD4+ T cells differentiate into helper T cells, which help to activate other immune cells, including B cells.

B cell activation, like T cell activation, requires antigen recognition. B cells express antibodies on their surface, which act as antigen receptors. When a B cell encounters an antigen that its antibody can bind to, the antigen is internalized and processed. The processed antigen is then presented on MHC class II molecules to helper T cells. The helper T cells provide the necessary signals to activate the B cell, leading to proliferation and differentiation. Some B cells differentiate into plasma cells, which are antibody-producing factories. These plasma cells secrete large quantities of antibodies that are specific for the antigen that initially activated the B cell. Other B cells differentiate into memory B cells, which provide long-lasting immunity. These memory B cells can quickly respond to future encounters with the same antigen, providing a faster and more effective immune response.

Antibodies, also known as immunoglobulins, are the key mediators of humoral immunity. They come in several different classes, each with distinct functions. IgG is the most abundant antibody in the blood and plays a major role in neutralizing pathogens, activating complement, and opsonizing pathogens for phagocytosis. IgM is the first antibody produced during an immune response and is particularly effective at activating complement. IgA is found in mucosal secretions, such as saliva and tears, and provides protection against pathogens at mucosal surfaces. IgE is involved in allergic reactions and also plays a role in defense against parasitic worms. Antibodies can neutralize pathogens by binding to them and preventing them from infecting cells. They can also opsonize pathogens, making them more easily recognized and engulfed by phagocytes. In addition, antibodies can activate the complement system, a cascade of proteins that leads to the destruction of pathogens.

The adaptive immune response is not just about clearing the infection; it's also about establishing immunological memory. This memory allows the immune system to respond more quickly and effectively to future encounters with the same pathogen. Memory T cells and memory B cells are long-lived cells that are specifically programmed to recognize the pathogen. Upon re-exposure to the pathogen, these memory cells are rapidly activated, leading to a faster and stronger immune response. This immunological memory is the basis of vaccination, which involves exposing the immune system to a weakened or inactive form of the pathogen to induce a memory response. Understanding the intricate details of the adaptive immune response is crucial for developing effective strategies to combat infectious diseases. By targeting specific steps in the immune response, researchers can design therapies that enhance immunity, prevent disease, or treat infections. For instance, vaccines can be designed to elicit strong antibody and T cell responses, providing long-lasting protection against specific pathogens. Immunomodulatory therapies can be used to dampen excessive inflammation or boost immune responses in individuals with weakened immune systems.

2 Chapter 2: Viral Entry Mechanisms

Gaining access to a host cell is the first critical step for any virus intending to replicate and propagate. This initial interaction, however, is far from a simple docking procedure. It's a sophisticated molecular dance, a lock-and-key engagement between viral surface proteins and specific receptors residing on the host cell's membrane. The precise nature of this interaction dictates the host range of the virus – determining which species, and even which cell types within a species, it can infect. A deep understanding of these receptor-binding dynamics is, therefore, paramount for crafting targeted antiviral strategies. Different viruses employ markedly different approaches to this attachment phase. Some, like the influenza virus, utilize hemagglutinin (HA) to bind to sialic acid residues ubiquitously present on many cell surfaces. Others, such as

HIV, require a more complex interaction involving the sequential binding to CD4 and then a co-receptor like CCR5 or CXCR4 on immune cells. This dual receptor requirement explains, in part, the tropism of HIV for specific immune cell populations. Furthermore, the affinity of the virus for its receptor, the number of receptors present on the cell surface, and the distribution of these receptors all influence the efficiency of viral entry. This intricate interplay of factors highlights the challenges involved in developing broadly effective antiviral therapies targeting this initial binding event. I think that researchers must be able to dissect these interactions at the molecular level using techniques like cryo-electron microscopy and surface plasmon resonance to visualize the structures of viral proteins bound to their receptors and to quantify the strength of these interactions. Such detailed knowledge is essential for rational drug design and for identifying novel therapeutic targets.

Following the initial receptor binding, the virus must then breach the cellular membrane to deliver its genetic material into the host cell's cytoplasm. Enveloped viruses, those surrounded by a lipid membrane derived from a previous host cell, typically achieve this through membrane fusion. This process involves the merging of the viral envelope with a host cell membrane, either at the cell surface or within an endosomal compartment. The driving force behind membrane fusion is the conformational change of viral fusion proteins, triggered by receptor binding or by the acidic environment within endosomes. For example, the influenza virus's HA protein undergoes a dramatic conformational change upon exposure to low pH in the endosome, exposing a hydrophobic fusion peptide that inserts into the target membrane. This insertion then pulls the viral and cellular membranes together, ultimately leading to fusion and release of the viral genome. Similarly, HIV's gp41 protein mediates fusion after gp120 binds to CD4 and a co-receptor. The precise mechanism of fusion can vary depending on the virus and the cell type. Some viruses fuse directly at the cell surface at neutral pH, while others require endocytosis followed by fusion within endosomes. Understanding these fusion pathways is crucial because they present attractive targets for antiviral intervention. Fusion inhibitors, such as enfuvirtide for HIV, directly block the conformational changes of fusion proteins, preventing membrane merger and viral entry. The development of effective fusion inhibitors requires detailed knowledge of the structure and function of viral fusion proteins, as well as the mechanisms that trigger their activation. Furthermore, resistance to fusion inhibitors can emerge through mutations in the viral fusion protein, underscoring the need for ongoing research and development of new generations of these drugs.

Non-enveloped viruses, lacking a lipid envelope, cannot fuse directly with the host cell membrane. Instead, they rely on endocytosis, a process by which the cell engulfs the virus within a vesicle. This endocytic pathway, normally used for nutrient uptake and cellular communication, is cleverly exploited by viruses to gain entry into the cell. Different viruses utilize different types of endocytosis, including clathrin-mediated endocytosis, caveolae-mediated endocytosis, and macropinocytosis. The choice of endocytic pathway often depends on the specific receptors used by the virus and the cell type it infects. For instance, some viruses induce receptor clustering on the cell surface, triggering clathrin-mediated endocytosis. Once inside the endosome, the virus must then escape to deliver its genome to the cytoplasm. This escape can involve disruption of the endosomal membrane, release of viral proteins that facilitate membrane penetration, or even direct translocation of the viral genome across the endosomal membrane. Adenoviruses, for example, disrupt the endosomal membrane using viral proteins, leading to the release of the virus into the cytoplasm. Other viruses, such as poliovirus, create pores in the endosomal membrane, allowing the viral RNA to enter the cytoplasm. The pH of the endosome plays a critical role in these escape mechanisms. As the endosome matures, its pH becomes increasingly acidic, triggering conformational changes in viral proteins that facilitate membrane disruption or pore formation. Inhibiting endosomal acidification with drugs like chloroquine can, in some cases, block viral entry by preventing these pH-dependent conformational changes. The endocytic pathway represents a complex and dynamic cellular process, and viruses have evolved sophisticated strategies to hijack this machinery for their own benefit. Targeting these processes with antiviral therapies is challenging, but the potential for broad-spectrum antiviral activity makes it a promising area of research. Understanding the specific endocytic pathways used by different viruses, the mechanisms by which they escape the endosome, and the role of endosomal pH in these processes is essential for developing effective antiviral strategies.

2.1 Receptor Binding Dynamics

Receptor binding isn't merely the first step in a viral infection; it's a carefully orchestrated molecular dance that dictates the virus's host range, tissue tropism, and overall infectivity. Understanding the nuances of this interaction is crucial for designing effective antiviral therapies. Viral attachment proteins (VAPs), studded on the viral surface, are responsible for initiating this interaction with specific receptors on the host cell membrane. These receptors are not randomly selected; they are typically proteins involved in essential cellular functions, making them readily accessible and abundant on the cell surface. This exploitation of normal cellular components is a hallmark of viral strategy.

The specificity of receptor binding is determined by the complementary shapes and chemical properties of the VAP and its cognate receptor. This interaction is governed by a combination of forces, including electrostatic interactions, hydrogen bonds, and van der Waals forces. Even subtle changes in the amino acid sequence of the VAP or the glycosylation pattern of the receptor can significantly alter the binding affinity, dictating whether infection can proceed. Consider, for example, the influenza virus hemagglutinin (HA) protein, which binds to sialic acid residues on host cell glycoproteins. Minor mutations in the HA protein can alter its affinity for different sialic acid linkages, influencing the virus's ability to infect avian versus human cells, a key factor in the emergence of pandemic strains. Beyond simple binding, the dynamics of receptor interaction are equally crucial. It's not just about whether a virus can bind to a receptor, but also how strongly and for how long. The association rate (kon) and dissociation rate (koff) of the VAP-receptor complex determine the overall binding affinity (Kd). A virus with a high kon and a low koff will exhibit a strong binding affinity, increasing the likelihood of successful infection. Furthermore, the stability of the receptor-virus interaction is also crucial, since the host cell's ability to clear or neutralize the virus is highly dependent on its characteristics. Think of it like trying to grab a slippery fish: a firm, lasting grip is far more effective than a fleeting touch.

The host cell receptor itself is not a passive player in this interaction. Many receptors are signaling molecules that trigger downstream cellular events upon ligand binding. Viruses can exploit these signaling pathways to facilitate their entry, replication, or immune evasion. For instance, some viruses trigger receptor-mediated endocytosis, a process where the virus is internalized into the cell within a vesicle. This provides a protected environment for the virus to uncoat and release its genetic material. Other viruses may trigger signaling pathways that suppress the host's immune response, creating a more permissive environment for viral replication. The human immunodeficiency virus (HIV), for example, binds to the CD4 receptor and the co-receptor CCR5 or CXCR4 on T cells, initiating a cascade of signaling events that ultimately lead to viral entry and T cell activation.

Furthermore, the distribution and density of receptors on the host cell surface can also influence viral infectivity. Cells with a high density of receptors are generally more susceptible to infection. Additionally, the spatial arrangement of receptors can play a role in viral entry. Some viruses require multiple receptors to cluster together on the cell surface to initiate entry, a process known as receptor clustering. This clustering can be facilitated by specific lipid rafts or other membrane microdomains.

Targeting receptor binding is an attractive strategy for antiviral drug development. One approach is to design small molecules that directly bind to the viral attachment protein, preventing it from interacting with its receptor. These molecules act as competitive inhibitors, effectively blocking the virus's entry into the cell. Another approach is to develop decoy receptors, soluble versions of the host cell receptor that bind to the virus in the extracellular space, preventing it from infecting cells. For example, the drug enfuvirtide targets the HIV gp41 protein, preventing it from fusing with the host cell membrane. Another approach involves antibodies that specifically target the viral attachment protein, neutralizing its ability to bind to its receptor.

However, viruses are masters of adaptation. They can rapidly evolve to escape the effects of antiviral drugs by mutating their viral attachment proteins. This is particularly true for viruses with high mutation rates, such as HIV and influenza virus. Therefore, it is crucial to develop antiviral strategies that target conserved regions of the viral attachment protein or that target multiple steps in the viral entry process.

In addition to drug development, understanding receptor binding dynamics is also essential for vaccine development. Vaccines often aim to elicit antibodies that neutralize the virus's ability to bind to its receptor. By understanding the specific epitopes (regions on the viral attachment protein) that are targeted by neutralizing antibodies, researchers can design more effective vaccines that elicit a strong and long-lasting immune response. This is often performed by measuring the virus' ability to attach to its receptor in the presence of patient's serum after vaccination.

Ultimately, deciphering the intricate dance of receptor binding dynamics is essential for combating emerging infectious disease agents. By gaining a deeper understanding of the molecular mechanisms that govern this interaction, we can develop more effective antiviral therapies and vaccines that prevent viral entry and protect us from the threat of viral infections. This knowledge needs to be constantly updated, because evolution pushes the virus to change and adapt for better survival.

2.2 Membrane Fusion Pathways

Membrane fusion is a fundamental process in biology, essential for everything from fertilization to neurotransmission, and, crucially, for the entry of many enveloped viruses into host cells. Unlike non-enveloped viruses that must disrupt the cell membrane to release their genome, enveloped viruses exploit the cell's own machinery to fuse their viral envelope with a host cell membrane, delivering their genetic material directly into the cytoplasm. This process is complex, tightly regulated, and a prime target for antiviral intervention. A crucial aspect of membrane fusion lies in its inherent energetic barrier. Membranes, composed primarily of phospholipids, naturally repel each other due to their charged head groups. Overcoming this repulsion requires a significant input of energy, typically provided by specialized fusion proteins. These proteins undergo dramatic conformational changes, bringing the two membranes into close proximity and facilitating the mixing of lipids, which ultimately leads to the formation of a continuous bilayer.

The precise mechanisms of membrane fusion vary depending on the virus and the host cell, but several common themes emerge. One of the most critical steps is receptor binding. Viruses utilize surface glycoproteins to bind to specific receptors on the host cell. This interaction is highly specific, determining which cell types a virus can infect, known as its tropism. Receptor binding triggers conformational changes in the viral fusion protein, initiating the fusion process. These receptors can vary widely in their molecular nature, ranging from proteins, such as CD4 for HIV, to carbohydrate moieties like sialic acid for influenza viruses. The binding affinity and subsequent activation of the fusion protein are critical determinants of viral infectivity.

Class I fusion proteins are characterized by a distinctive alpha-helical structure and undergo substantial conformational changes during fusion, inserting a fusion peptide into the target membrane. Influenza virus hemagglutinin

(HA) is a classic example. HA is synthesized as a precursor protein that must be cleaved by host cell proteases into HA1 and HA2 subunits. This cleavage is essential for infectivity, as it exposes the fusion peptide within HA2. Upon binding to sialic acid receptors and exposure to the acidic environment of the endosome, HA undergoes a dramatic conformational rearrangement, extending the fusion peptide towards the target membrane. The fusion peptide then inserts into the host cell membrane, initiating the fusion process. The refolding of HA pulls the viral and cellular membranes together, leading to hemifusion, where the outer leaflets of the two membranes merge, followed by the formation of a fusion pore and release of the viral genome. A similar mechanism is employed by HIV's gp41. Class II fusion proteins, found in flaviviruses like dengue and Zika, employ a different mechanism. These proteins are typically arranged as dimers on the viral surface and undergo a "lying-down" conformational change upon triggering. Unlike Class I proteins, they do not require acidic pH for activation but rely on receptor binding and subsequent conformational rearrangements. Fusion is initiated by the insertion of a hydrophobic loop into the target membrane, followed by refolding that brings the viral and cellular membranes into close apposition. This process is less reliant on dramatic helical refolding compared to Class I proteins but still requires precise coordination and significant energy input.

Class III fusion proteins, exemplified by those found in vesicular stomatitis virus (VSV), share characteristics of both Class I and Class II proteins. They exhibit large-scale conformational changes and often require low pH for activation. These proteins mediate fusion through a complex series of steps, involving receptor binding, triggering by low pH, and insertion of a fusion peptide or loop into the target membrane. The exact details of the fusion mechanism for Class III proteins are still under investigation, highlighting the diversity and complexity of membrane fusion processes.

The location where fusion occurs – at the cell surface or within endosomes – is also a critical factor. Some viruses, like HIV, can fuse directly with the plasma membrane at neutral pH, allowing for rapid entry into the cell. Others, such as influenza, are internalized via endocytosis and fuse with the endosomal membrane after exposure to acidic pH. This pH-dependent fusion is a clever strategy employed by the virus to ensure fusion occurs only after the virus has been safely internalized and is not exposed to the extracellular environment. The acidic pH triggers conformational changes in the fusion protein, leading to its activation and subsequent membrane fusion.

Understanding the intricacies of membrane fusion pathways is crucial for developing effective antiviral therapies. Fusion inhibitors are a class of drugs that target viral fusion proteins, preventing them from mediating membrane fusion and blocking viral entry. Enfuvirtide, an HIV fusion inhibitor, is a synthetic peptide that mimics a region of gp41, preventing it from undergoing the conformational changes necessary for fusion. Maraviroc is another antiretroviral drug that targets the host cell receptor CCR5, blocking HIV from binding and entering the cell. Other potential therapeutic strategies include developing antibodies that neutralize viral fusion proteins or targeting host cell factors that are essential for fusion.

Furthermore, targeting the endocytic pathway can also prevent infection, because of the implications that some viruses have to depend on this pathway.

The development of new antiviral therapies targeting membrane fusion requires a detailed understanding of the structural biology of viral fusion proteins and the cellular factors involved in the fusion process. Cryo-electron microscopy and X-ray crystallography have provided invaluable insights into the structure of these proteins and the conformational changes they undergo during fusion. These insights are crucial for designing drugs that specifically target the fusion process and block viral entry.

In summary, membrane fusion is a complex and highly regulated process that is essential for the entry of enveloped viruses into host cells. Understanding the different types of fusion proteins, the mechanisms of fusion, and the cellular factors involved is crucial for developing effective antiviral therapies. By targeting the fusion process, we can block viral entry and prevent infection, contributing to the development of new strategies for combating emerging infectious diseases. The continued research in this area holds great promise for the development of novel antiviral agents that can effectively target a broad range of viral infections.

2.3 Endocytic Route Exploitation

The cellular world, a bustling metropolis of activity, provides multiple points of entry for viruses. While direct fusion with the plasma membrane is a straightforward route for some, many viruses cleverly exploit the cell's natural endocytic pathways to gain access. This is no passive process; viruses actively manipulate these pathways to ensure their survival and replication. Understanding these mechanisms is crucial for designing effective antiviral therapies.

Endocytosis, a fundamental process for cells to internalize extracellular material, comes in various flavors, each with distinct characteristics and susceptibilities to viral hijacking. Clathrin-mediated endocytosis, perhaps the best-studied, involves the assembly of a protein coat, primarily clathrin, at the plasma membrane to form vesicles that bud inward, carrying cargo molecules. Caveolae-mediated endocytosis, on the other hand, utilizes small, flask-shaped invaginations of the plasma membrane enriched in caveolins and other proteins. Macropinocytosis, often triggered by growth factors or other stimuli, involves the formation of large, irregular membrane ruffles that engulf extracellular fluid and particles. Still others, such as clathrin\item and caveolae-independent endocytosis, exist as well and also use various mechanisms of action that are still not completely understood. Viruses have evolved elegant strategies to exploit one or more of these endocytic routes, often tailoring their entry pathway to specific cell types and host species.

How do viruses actually take control? The process often starts with viral binding to cell surface receptors. Many viruses bind to receptors specifically found in clathrin-coated pits, naturally drawing them towards that endocytic pathway. However, the simple binding is not enough. The virus must send signals to the host cell's machinery. For example, many viruses use interactions with adapter proteins, such as AP-2, to promote their incorporation into clathrin-coated vesicles. These adapter proteins bridge the gap between viral surface proteins and the clathrin coat, effectively recruiting the virus into the endocytic machinery. However, hijacking caveolae or inducing macropinocytosis also relies on specific signal transduction pathways that viruses can activate via receptor binding or direct membrane interactions. Viruses can trigger a cascade of signaling events that lead to the assembly of caveolae or the formation of macropinocytic cups, essentially tricking the cell into engulfing them.

Once inside the endosome, the virus faces another hurdle: escaping degradation within the lysosome, a cellular organelle filled with digestive enzymes. This is where the acidification of the endosome becomes a critical factor. As the endosome matures, its internal pH drops, creating an acidic environment. Many viruses have evolved acid-activated fusion proteins that trigger membrane fusion between the viral envelope and the endosomal membrane. This fusion event releases the viral genome into the cytoplasm, allowing the virus to begin replication. The timing is crucial; premature fusion could lead to the virus being trapped in the wrong cellular compartment, while delayed fusion could result in degradation.

To accomplish this, viruses have evolved mechanisms to delay endosomal maturation, effectively creating a more hospitable environment for their escape. Some viruses interfere with the trafficking of endosomes, preventing them from fusing with lysosomes. Others actively disrupt lysosomal function, reducing their ability to degrade viral components. The endocytic pathway can be exploited to transport the viral particle near specific organelles, like the endoplasmic reticulum.

Consider, for example, the influenza virus, a master of endocytic entry. It binds to sialic acid receptors on the cell surface and is internalized via clathrin-mediated endocytosis. The acidic environment of the endosome triggers a conformational change in the hemagglutinin (HA) protein, a viral surface glycoprotein. This conformational change exposes a fusion peptide that inserts into the endosomal membrane, initiating membrane fusion and releasing the viral RNA into the cytoplasm. Similarly, certain picornaviruses exploit the macropinocytosis pathway. These viruses trigger the formation of large membrane ruffles that engulf them, allowing them to enter the cell in a non-selective manner. Once inside the macropinosome, the virus disrupts the normal maturation process, preventing fusion with lysosomes and creating a protected environment for replication.

The implications of understanding these viral entry mechanisms are significant. By targeting specific steps in the endocytic pathway, we can develop novel antiviral therapies. For instance, drugs that block viral receptor binding can prevent the initial entry of the virus into the cell. Inhibitors of endosomal acidification can prevent the triggering of fusion proteins, trapping the virus within the endosome. Alternatively, drugs that interfere with viral trafficking or disrupt lysosomal function can also inhibit viral replication.

Beyond direct inhibition of viral entry, modulating the host cell's endocytic machinery itself presents another avenue for therapeutic intervention. By targeting specific host cell proteins involved in endocytosis, we can indirectly block viral entry and replication. For example, inhibitors of dynamin, a GTPase essential for vesicle scission, can prevent the formation of endocytic vesicles, effectively blocking viral entry. However, such interventions must be carefully considered, as they can also disrupt normal cellular function.

There is still much to learn about the complex interplay between viruses and the endocytic pathway. New research is continuously unveiling novel mechanisms by which viruses manipulate these pathways, leading to new therapeutic targets. As our understanding of these processes grows, we will be better equipped to combat viral infections and develop more effective antiviral therapies. I, for one, am hopeful that future discoveries will lead to more robust and specific antiviral strategies. The future of medicine rests on a deeper comprehension of how infectious agents manipulate these cellular processes and our creativity to exploit those weaknesses for the benefit of our health. The road ahead is challenging, but the potential rewards are immense.

3 Chapter 3: Bacterial Invasion Strategies

Bacterial invasion is a multifaceted process, not a single event. It requires a carefully orchestrated series of events for a bacterium to successfully breach host defenses, establish a foothold, and ultimately, cause disease. It is a dance of molecular interactions, driven by bacterial virulence factors and countered by host immune responses.

Adhesion is the initial and critical step. Think of it as a bacterium trying to stick to a slippery surface. To succeed, it employs specialized structures known as adhesins. These are often located on pili (hair-like appendages) or directly on the bacterial cell surface. Adhesins are like molecular Velcro, recognizing and binding to specific receptors on host cells. These receptors can be proteins, carbohydrates, or lipids – essentially any molecule displayed on the cell surface that provides a good grip for the adhesin. The specificity of this interaction is crucial. Certain bacteria can only infect specific tissues or cell types because they express adhesins that only recognize receptors found in those locations. For instance, Escherichia coli strains that cause urinary tract infections express adhesins that bind specifically to receptors on the surface of bladder epithelial cells. Blocking these adhesins with specific antibodies or other molecules is being explored as a potential therapeutic strategy to prevent infection. However, adhesion alone is not enough. Bacteria also need to overcome the constant washing away action of bodily fluids and the physical barrier of the mucus layer that lines many tissues. This is where biofilm formation comes into play. Biofilms are complex communities of bacteria encased in a self-produced matrix of extracellular polymeric substances (EPS). Think of it as a bacterial fortress, protecting the bacteria from antibiotics, disinfectants, and host immune cells. Colonization, the establishment of a bacterial population at a specific site, is often facilitated by biofilm formation. These biofilms can be incredibly difficult to eradicate, contributing to chronic infections.

Toxins are like weapons in the bacterial arsenal. They represent a diverse array of molecules that can damage host cells and disrupt normal cellular function. Some toxins are secreted directly into the surrounding environment (exotoxins), while others are released only upon bacterial cell lysis (endotoxins). Exotoxins, in particular, exhibit a wide range of activities. Some, like diphtheria toxin produced by Corynebacterium diphtheriae, act as enzymes that modify and inactivate essential cellular proteins, leading to cell death. Others, like cholera toxin produced by Vibrio cholerae, disrupt ion transport across cell membranes, causing massive fluid loss and diarrhea. Then there are toxins that target specific cell types, such as neurotoxins produced by Clostridium botulinum and Clostridium tetani, which interfere with nerve function, causing paralysis. Superantigens, like toxic shock syndrome toxin-1 (TSST-1) produced by Staphylococcus aureus, are a unique class of exotoxins that bypass normal antigen processing and directly stimulate a massive T cell response. This can lead to a cytokine storm, a life-threatening condition characterized by excessive inflammation and organ damage. Understanding the specific mechanisms of action of bacterial toxins is crucial for developing effective antitoxins and other therapies that can neutralize their harmful effects.

Invasion of host cells is another critical strategy employed by many pathogenic bacteria. This goes beyond simple adhesion and involves the bacterium actively entering and residing within the host cell. Some bacteria, like Salmonella and Shigella, induce host cells to engulf them through a process called induced endocytosis. They inject effector proteins into the host cell, which manipulate the cytoskeleton (the cell's internal scaffolding) to create membrane ruffles that engulf the bacterium. Other bacteria, like Listeria monocytogenes, can directly penetrate host cells using specialized surface proteins called internalins. Once inside the host cell, bacteria can either remain within a vacuole (a membrane-bound compartment) or escape into the cytoplasm. Salmonella, for example, remains within a modified vacuole, where it can replicate and spread to other cells. Listeria, on the other hand, escapes from the vacuole and replicates directly in the cytoplasm, moving from cell to cell by polymerizing actin filaments into a "rocket" that propels the bacterium forward. This intracellular lifestyle provides bacteria with protection from extracellular immune defenses and access to nutrients, allowing them to establish a persistent infection.

Furthermore, quorum sensing adds a layer of complexity to bacterial invasion. Bacteria are not solitary creatures. They communicate with each other using small signaling molecules called autoinducers. When the concentration of these autoinducers reaches a certain threshold (a "quorum"), it triggers a coordinated change in gene expression, affecting a wide range of bacterial behaviors, including virulence factor production, biofilm formation, and even invasion. This allows bacteria to act as a collective, optimizing their strategies for survival and infection. Inhibiting quorum sensing is being explored as a novel approach to combat bacterial infections, disrupting their coordinated attack and rendering them more susceptible to host defenses. I think targeting quorum sensing can make the bacterias alone and unable to perform the coordinated attack.

The battle between bacteria and their host is a constant evolutionary arms race. Bacteria are constantly evolving new strategies to invade and exploit host cells, while hosts are developing new defenses to counteract these attacks. Understanding the intricate details of bacterial invasion strategies is essential for developing effective therapies to prevent and treat infectious diseases. By targeting specific bacterial virulence factors, disrupting bacterial communication, and boosting host immune responses, we can gain the upper hand in this ongoing conflict.

3.1 Adhesion and Colonization

Adhesion and colonization represent the initial and pivotal steps in bacterial pathogenesis. Without successful attachment to host tissues, most bacteria are simply cleared by natural defense mechanisms, like the mucociliary escalator in the respiratory tract or peristalsis in the gut. Colonization, the subsequent proliferation and establishment of a bacterial population at the site of adhesion, is equally crucial for initiating infection and disease. Both processes are intricate, involving a complex interplay of bacterial factors, host receptors, and environmental conditions. Therefore understanding them is key to developing targeted antimicrobial strategies.

Bacterial adhesion is not a passive process. It relies on specialized structures called adhesins, which are surface molecules, often proteins or carbohydrates, displayed on the bacterial cell wall, pili, fimbriae, or even within the extracellular matrix. These adhesins exhibit remarkable specificity, binding to complementary receptors on host cell surfaces. These host receptors can be a diverse range of molecules, including glycoproteins, glycolipids, integrins, and other cell surface proteins. The interaction between a bacterial adhesin and a host receptor acts like a lock and key, determining which tissues a particular bacterium can infect. For example, Escherichia coli strains that cause urinary tract infections (UTIs) express P-fimbriae with adhesins that specifically bind to glycolipids on the surface of uroepithelial cells, explaining their propensity to infect the urinary tract. The strength and nature of the adhesion also play significant roles, ranging from weak, reversible interactions that allow bacteria to explore the surface, to strong, irreversible attachments that anchor them firmly in place. Moreover, this initial attachment can trigger signaling cascades within the host cell, further facilitating bacterial invasion or modulating the immune response.

Following initial adhesion, successful colonization hinges on a bacterium's ability to overcome host defenses and acquire essential nutrients for survival and replication. The host body is not a passive environment; it actively resists colonization through various mechanisms. These include the continuous shedding of epithelial cells, the flow of bodily fluids, the presence of antimicrobial substances like lysozyme and defensins, and the constant surveillance by the immune system. To counter these challenges, bacteria employ diverse strategies. One strategy is the production of biofilms, complex communities of bacteria encased in a self-produced matrix of extracellular polymeric substances (EPS). Biofilms provide a protective shield against antibiotics, disinfectants, and the host's immune cells, making them notoriously difficult to eradicate. They also enable bacteria to adhere more strongly to surfaces and to each other, facilitating long-term colonization. Nutrient acquisition is also paramount. Bacteria must compete with host cells for essential nutrients like iron, zinc, and amino acids. They often produce siderophores, high-affinity iron-chelating molecules, to scavenge iron from the host environment. Other bacteria secrete enzymes that degrade complex molecules into simpler, more readily available nutrients. Furthermore, bacteria can adapt their metabolism to utilize available resources efficiently.

However, the local environment significantly influences adhesion and colonization. pH, temperature, oxygen levels, and the presence of other microorganisms can all impact bacterial growth and behavior. Some bacteria thrive in acidic conditions, while others prefer alkaline environments. Temperature affects the expression of bacterial genes, including those encoding adhesins and virulence factors. Anaerobic bacteria colonize oxygen-depleted environments, while aerobic bacteria require oxygen for growth. The presence of other microorganisms can also be a major factor. Some bacteria compete with each other for resources, while others form synergistic relationships, enhancing each other's colonization abilities. These interactions can be complex and dynamic, shaping the overall composition of the microbial community.

The implications of understanding bacterial adhesion and colonization are far-reaching. By identifying the specific adhesins and host receptors involved in these processes, researchers can develop targeted therapeutics to disrupt bacterial attachment and prevent infection. These strategies include designing drugs that block adhesin-receptor interactions, developing antibodies that neutralize adhesins, or creating vaccines that elicit an immune response against adhesins. Furthermore, understanding the mechanisms by which bacteria overcome host defenses and colonize tissues can lead to novel approaches for preventing and treating infections. For instance, strategies that disrupt biofilm formation, enhance nutrient competition, or modulate the host's immune response could prove highly effective.

Adhesion and colonization mechanisms vary dramatically across different bacterial species. Streptococcus pneumoniae, a leading cause of pneumonia, uses phosphorylcholine on its surface to bind to platelet-activating factor receptor (PAFR) on lung cells. This interaction promotes internalization into the host cell. Vibrio cholerae, the causative agent of cholera, employs toxin-coregulated pili (TCP) to adhere to the intestinal epithelium. The expression of TCP is tightly regulated by environmental conditions, such as pH and temperature, in the gut. Staphylococcus aureus, a highly versatile pathogen, expresses a variety of adhesins, including microbial surface components recognizing adhesive matrix molecules (MSCRAMMs), which bind to components of the extracellular matrix, like fibronectin and collagen, facilitating colonization of various tissues. Pseudomonas aeruginosa, known for its ability to form biofilms, uses type IV pili for initial attachment, followed by the production of alginate, an extracellular polysaccharide, to create a robust biofilm matrix.

Finally, preventing bacterial adhesion and colonization is an evolving field with innovative technologies paving the way. Anti-adhesion therapies are being actively explored as potential alternatives or adjuncts to traditional antibiotics. These therapies aim to neutralize bacterial adhesins or block their interaction with host receptors, preventing the initial attachment and subsequent colonization. Phage therapy utilizes bacteriophages, viruses that infect and kill bacteria, to target specific pathogens and disrupt their colonization. Immunomodulatory approaches focus on enhancing the host's natural defenses to prevent or control bacterial colonization. These strategies include stimulating the production of antimicrobial peptides, strengthening the epithelial barrier, or modulating the immune response to promote bacterial clearance. Probiotics, live microorganisms that confer a health benefit on the host, can also be used to prevent bacterial colonization by competing with pathogens for resources and adhesion sites.

3.2 Toxin-Mediated Damage

Toxins are potent weapons in the bacterial arsenal, serving as pivotal mediators of damage during infection. These molecules, often proteins or lipopolysaccharides, directly interact with host cells, disrupting normal cellular processes and triggering a cascade of events that ultimately lead to tissue injury and disease manifestation. Understanding the diverse array of bacterial toxins and their mechanisms of action is paramount to developing effective therapeutic strategies.

Some bacteria deploy exotoxins, secreted toxins that travel from the site of infection to exert their effects on distant tissues. One prominent example is diphtheria toxin, produced by Corynebacterium diphtheriae. This toxin gains entry into host cells via receptor-mediated endocytosis. Once inside, it inhibits protein synthesis by catalyzing the ADP-ribosylation of elongation factor 2 (EF-2), a critical component of the ribosome. This modification effectively halts protein production, leading to cell death and the characteristic pseudomembrane formation in the throat associated with diphtheria. The potency of diphtheria toxin underscores the devastating consequences of disrupting fundamental cellular processes.

Another class of exotoxins are the superantigens, exemplified by toxic shock syndrome toxin-1 (TSST-1) produced by Staphylococcus aureus. Unlike conventional antigens that require processing and presentation by antigen-presenting cells, superantigens directly bind to the major histocompatibility complex (MHC) class II molecules on antigen-presenting cells and T cell receptors, bypassing the normal antigen-specific activation pathway. This non-specific interaction triggers a massive T cell activation, resulting in the release of copious amounts of cytokines, including interleukin-1 (IL-1), tumor necrosis factor-alpha (TNF-), and interferon-gamma (IFN-). The resulting "cytokine storm" leads to systemic inflammation, fever, shock, and potentially multi-organ failure, as seen in toxic shock syndrome. The systemic nature of superantigen-mediated damage highlights the importance of understanding the broader immunological consequences of toxin exposure.

In contrast to exotoxins, endotoxins are structural components of the bacterial cell wall, most notably lipopolysaccharide (LPS) found in Gram-negative bacteria. LPS is released upon bacterial lysis or during active bacterial growth. When LPS enters the bloodstream, it binds to LPS-binding protein (LBP), which then delivers it to CD14 on the surface of immune cells, particularly macrophages. This interaction triggers the activation of Toll-like receptor 4 (TLR4), a pattern recognition receptor that initiates intracellular signaling cascades. These pathways ultimately lead to the activation of NF-B, a transcription factor that promotes the expression of pro-inflammatory cytokines. The resulting cytokine production contributes to systemic inflammation, fever, hypotension, disseminated intravascular coagulation (DIC), and potentially septic shock. The cascade of events initiated by LPS demonstrates how a structural component of the bacterial cell can induce a potent and potentially lethal inflammatory response.

Beyond these broad categories, many bacteria produce toxins that target specific cellular components or processes. For instance, Clostridium botulinum produces botulinum toxin, a potent neurotoxin that blocks the release of acetylcholine at neuromuscular junctions. This blockade prevents muscle contraction, leading to flaccid paralysis. The exquisite specificity of botulinum toxin for neuronal targets highlights the potential for targeted therapies, as evidenced by its use in treating neurological disorders and cosmetic applications.

Furthermore, Vibrio cholerae produces cholera toxin, which disrupts ion transport in intestinal epithelial cells. This toxin ADP-ribosylates a G protein, leading to constitutive activation of adenylate cyclase and increased levels of cyclic AMP (cAMP). Elevated cAMP levels stimulate the secretion of chloride ions and inhibit the absorption of sodium ions, resulting in massive water efflux from the cells and the characteristic profuse watery diarrhea associated with cholera. The disruption of intestinal homeostasis by cholera toxin underscores the importance of maintaining proper ion balance for normal physiological function.

Combating toxin-mediated damage requires a multifaceted approach. One strategy involves the use of antitoxins, which are antibodies that neutralize the activity of the toxin. Antitoxins are typically produced by immunizing animals with inactivated toxins or toxoids. The resulting antibodies bind to the toxin, preventing it from interacting with host cells and thereby neutralizing its harmful effects. Antitoxins have been successfully used to treat diphtheria, tetanus, and botulism.

Another approach focuses on developing drugs that inhibit toxin production or activity. For example, several compounds are being investigated for their ability to inhibit the secretion of bacterial toxins. Other strategies aim to block the interaction of toxins with host cell receptors or to interfere with the intracellular signaling pathways activated by toxins. The development of such drugs requires a detailed understanding of the molecular mechanisms of toxin action.

Additionally, supportive care plays a crucial role in managing toxin-mediated diseases. This includes maintaining fluid and electrolyte balance, providing respiratory support, and managing complications such as septic shock and organ failure. In severe cases, dialysis or other organ support therapies may be necessary.

In summary, toxin-mediated damage is a significant mechanism of bacterial pathogenesis. Understanding the diverse array of bacterial toxins, their mechanisms of action, and the host responses they elicit is essential for developing effective therapeutic strategies. A multifaceted approach, combining antitoxins, drugs that inhibit toxin production or activity, and supportive care, is often necessary to combat the devastating effects of bacterial toxins.

4 Chapter 4: Intracellular Trafficking Hijack

Once inside the cell, pathogens don't simply sit idly by; they actively manipulate the host's internal transport systems, the intricate network of pathways that govern the movement of molecules and organelles. This subversion, known as intracellular trafficking hijack, is a critical element of their survival and replication strategy. Imagine the cell's interior as a bustling city, with a complex road system for delivering goods and disposing of waste. Infectious agents, with nefarious intent, reroute these pathways for their own purposes, effectively turning the city's infrastructure against its inhabitants.

The endosomal pathway, responsible for sorting and delivering cargo to lysosomes for degradation or recycling back to the cell surface, is a prime target. Many viruses and bacteria enter the cell through endocytosis, a process where the cell membrane invaginates to engulf the pathogen. Normally, the endosome would mature, becoming increasingly acidic and eventually fusing with a lysosome, where powerful enzymes break down the contents. However, savvy pathogens have evolved mechanisms to prevent this fate. Some viruses, for example, can block the acidification of the endosome, preventing the activation of lysosomal enzymes and ensuring their own survival. Others can escape the endosome altogether, releasing themselves into the cytoplasm, where they can begin replicating. This escape often involves the use of viral proteins that disrupt the endosomal membrane, creating pores through which the virus can pass. Bacterial pathogens might secrete effector proteins directly into the host cell cytoplasm that interfere with the normal maturation of endosomes. These bacterial effectors can recruit or block the recruitment of essential proteins that are important for vesicle trafficking and fusion, ultimately preventing the degradation of the bacteria within the endosome. Think of it as a burglar jamming the lock on a safe, preventing the authorities from accessing its contents.

Autophagy, another key cellular process, is also frequently targeted. This process, meaning "self-eating," is a survival mechanism where cells engulf damaged or unnecessary components, including pathogens, within double-membrane vesicles called autophagosomes. These autophagosomes then fuse with lysosomes, where the contents are degraded. However, many pathogens have developed ways to either inhibit autophagy or exploit it for their own benefit. Some viruses encode proteins that directly block the formation of autophagosomes, preventing the cell from clearing them. Others can redirect autophagy, using the autophagosomes as a safe haven for replication. In this scenario, the virus can replicate within the autophagosome, protected from the host's immune defenses. Similarly, some bacteria have evolved to manipulate autophagy. These bacteria can either block the formation of autophagosome, or they can even redirect them to create a protective niche for replication within the host cell. The pathogen essentially turns the cell's recycling system into a personal bodyguard and incubator.

The Golgi apparatus, the cell's central processing and packaging plant for proteins, is another important target. This organelle is responsible for modifying, sorting, and packaging proteins destined for secretion or delivery to other organelles. Viral infections frequently disrupt the Golgi network to enhance virus production and assembly. Some viruses disrupt the normal architecture of the Golgi, causing it to fragment or collapse. This disruption can interfere with the processing and trafficking of cellular proteins, but more importantly, it can redirect the Golgi's resources towards the production of viral proteins. For instance, viral proteins are often glycosylated in the Golgi, a process that is essential for their proper folding and function. By hijacking the Golgi, viruses can ensure that their proteins are correctly processed and packaged, maximizing their infectivity. In the case of bacteria, some bacterial toxins are able to modify key Golgi proteins, disrupting its ability to properly fold and traffic proteins. Furthermore, disruption of the Golgi apparatus may impair the secretion of cytokines, thereby dampening the host's immune response.

The consequences of intracellular trafficking hijack are far-reaching. By disrupting these pathways, pathogens can evade immune defenses, promote their replication, and ultimately cause disease. Understanding the molecular mechanisms underlying these hijacking strategies is essential for developing effective therapeutic interventions. Developing drugs that can restore normal trafficking pathways or prevent pathogens from manipulating them could represent a novel approach to treating infectious diseases. For example, molecules that enhance lysosomal function could promote the degradation of pathogens within endosomes and autophagosomes. Alternatively, compounds that disrupt the interaction between viral proteins and trafficking machinery could prevent viruses from hijacking these pathways. Developing a deep comprehension of the complex and intricate nature of intracellular trafficking is not just an academic exercise; it's a critical step in protecting ourselves from the ever-evolving threat of infectious diseases. I believe that future therapies may even be able to target multiple trafficking pathways simultaneously, offering a more comprehensive defense against a wide range of pathogens. The cellular world is like a battlefield, and intracellular trafficking is one of its most critical fronts.

4.1 Endosomal Pathway Subversion

Intracellular trafficking pathways represent a complex and dynamic network essential for cellular function, and microbes have evolved sophisticated strategies to exploit these routes for their own survival and propagation. A crucial aspect of this subversion centers around the endosomal pathway, a major route for internalizing extracellular material and regulating membrane protein trafficking. This intricate system, normally responsible for sort-

ing, modifying, and degrading internalized cargo, becomes a playground for pathogens seeking to establish infection and evade host defenses. The pathogens don't only hijack the endosomal pathway but, for example, they change the pH of it, leading to its deactivation.
The process typically begins with the pathogen gaining entry into the host cell via receptor-mediated endocytosis, a process that normally brings nutrients and signaling molecules into the cell. However, many viruses and bacteria have evolved surface proteins that mimic or directly interact with cellular receptors, triggering their own internalization. Once inside the endosome, these pathogens face a crucial decision point: escape the endosome before it fuses with lysosomes, where degradation occurs, or manipulate the endosomal environment to their advantage. For example, Listeria monocytogenes, a bacterium that causes foodborne illness, secretes a pore-forming toxin called listeriolysin O (LLO). LLO disrupts the endosomal membrane, allowing the bacteria to escape into the cytoplasm, where it can multiply freely. This escape strategy avoids the harsh conditions of the lysosome and allows the bacterium to access the nutrient-rich cytoplasm. On the other hand, some pathogens remain within the endosomal compartment but actively modify its characteristics

to create a replicative niche.

To maintain their intracellular sanctuary and facilitate replication, pathogens must interfere with the normal maturation and trafficking of endosomes. This often involves disrupting the endosomal sorting machinery, a complex network of proteins that directs cargo to different destinations within the cell. Rab proteins, a family of small GTPases, play a key role in regulating endosomal trafficking by controlling vesicle budding, motility, and fusion. Different Rab proteins are associated with distinct stages of endosome maturation, and pathogens can manipulate these proteins to alter the fate of their containing vesicles. For instance, some viruses recruit specific Rab proteins to their replication sites, creating a specialized compartment that supports viral replication and prevents degradation. Another strategy involves interfering with the fusion of endosomes with lysosomes. Lysosomes are the cell's primary degradative organelles, containing a variety of enzymes that break down proteins, lipids, and nucleic acids. Pathogens can prevent lysosomal fusion by disrupting the trafficking of lysosomal proteins, inhibiting the activity of lysosomal enzymes, or physically blocking the fusion process. By inhibiting lysosomal fusion, pathogens can prevent their own degradation and maintain a safe haven within the host cell.

Beyond simply surviving within the endosomal pathway, some pathogens actively exploit this system to spread throughout the host organism. This can involve manipulating endosomal trafficking to promote the release of pathogens from infected cells or to facilitate their transport to other cells. One mechanism involves hijacking the exosomal pathway, a process by which cells release small vesicles called exosomes that contain proteins, lipids, and nucleic acids. Pathogens can redirect their trafficking into exosomes, effectively using these vesicles as Trojan horses to infect neighboring cells. This strategy allows pathogens to spread without ever being exposed to the extracellular environment, evading the host's immune defenses. A quite famous family of proteins, the SNARE proteins, can be used by pathogens to promote or inhibit the release of pathogens from infected cells.

Understanding the intricate mechanisms by which pathogens subvert the endosomal pathway is crucial for developing new therapeutic strategies to combat infectious diseases. Targeting these pathways can disrupt pathogen replication, prevent their spread, and enhance the host's immune response. One approach is to develop drugs that interfere with the pathogen's ability to enter cells via endocytosis. These drugs could block the interaction between the pathogen and its host cell receptor, preventing internalization. Another approach is to target the pathogen's ability to manipulate endosomal trafficking. This could involve developing drugs that inhibit the activity of Rab proteins or disrupt the trafficking of lysosomal proteins. For example, drugs that restore normal lysosomal function could promote the degradation of pathogens within the endosomal pathway. Importantly, new strategies are aiming at stimulating immunity responses, such as activating NK cells.

The constant arms race between pathogens and their hosts has led to the evolution of remarkable adaptations on both sides. By understanding the intricate details of how pathogens subvert the endosomal pathway, we can develop new and effective strategies to combat infectious diseases. This ongoing research effort promises to provide innovative solutions for protecting human health against the ever-evolving threat of microbial pathogens. Further studies are ongoing to have more precise tools to fight these diseases, such as CRISPR editing and new immunization techniques.

4.2 Autophagy Interference

Autophagy, a highly conserved cellular process, plays a pivotal role in maintaining cellular homeostasis by degrading and recycling damaged organelles, misfolded proteins, and intracellular pathogens. It is a crucial defense mechanism against invading microorganisms, including viruses and bacteria. However, many infectious agents have evolved sophisticated strategies to interfere with autophagy, either to suppress its protective effects or to exploit it for their own replication and dissemination. This interference can significantly impact the course of infection and the host's ability to mount an effective immune response.

Pathogens interfere with autophagy at multiple stages, from initiation to degradation. A common strategy employed by some viruses involves blocking the formation of autophagosomes, the double-membraned vesicles that engulf cellular cargo destined for degradation. These viruses often encode proteins that directly interact with key autophagy regulators, such as Beclin 1, Atg5, or LC3, thereby disrupting the normal progression of autophagy. For instance, certain viral proteins can bind to Beclin 1, preventing its interaction with other proteins required for autophagosome nucleation. This effectively halts the initiation of autophagy, allowing the virus to replicate unchecked within the host cell. Others can target the Atg proteins, which are essential for autophagosome formation, directly reducing autophagosome number.

Another strategy used by pathogens is to redirect autophagosomes to promote their own replication. Instead of being degraded by autophagy, these pathogens are sequestered within autophagosomes that are then modified to create a protective niche for their replication. This can involve altering the fusion of autophagosomes with lysosomes, the cellular organelles responsible for degradation. Some viruses, for example, prevent the fusion of autophagosomes with lysosomes, preventing the degradation of their components, and converting the vesicles into replication compartments. In other cases, pathogens can actively promote the fusion of autophagosomes with other cellular compartments, such as endosomes or the endoplasmic reticulum, to acquire nutrients or to facilitate their egress from the cell. This exploitation of autophagy can significantly enhance pathogen replication and spread. This could lead to the increased production of viral particles, leading to more viruses escaping from the host cell.

Beyond blocking or redirecting autophagy, some pathogens actively degrade autophagy components. Viruses can encode proteases that specifically target key autophagy proteins, leading to their degradation and the suppression of autophagy. This degradation can occur through various mechanisms, including direct cleavage of autophagy proteins or by promoting their ubiquitination and subsequent degradation by the proteasome. By eliminating these essential autophagy components, pathogens can effectively cripple the host cell's ability to clear the infection. In the long run, the prolonged degradation of autophagy proteins may lead to the dysfunction of the autophagic pathways, making the host more vulnerable to future infections.

Furthermore, several bacteria species manipulate the autophagy pathway to establish long-term chronic infections. These intracellular bacteria have developed sophisticated mechanisms to either inhibit or stimulate autophagy depending on the stage of infection and their location within the host cell. For example, some bacteria initially trigger autophagy to facilitate their entry into host cells, but then quickly suppress autophagy to prevent their degradation. This can involve secreting effector proteins that interfere with autophagy signaling pathways or by modifying the autophagosome membrane to prevent its fusion with lysosomes. This careful control of autophagy allows these bacteria to survive and replicate within host cells for extended periods, contributing to chronic infection. Moreover, some bacteria can benefit from the host cell's metabolic support when they are located inside the autophagosome.

The consequences of autophagy interference by pathogens are far-reaching. By disrupting this crucial cellular process, pathogens can evade immune detection, enhance their replication, and promote cell survival. The suppression of autophagy can also lead to the accumulation of damaged organelles and misfolded proteins, contributing to cellular stress and inflammation. Chronic inflammation, in turn, can further compromise the host's immune response and promote the development of disease. Therefore, understanding how pathogens interfere with autophagy is essential for developing effective therapeutic strategies to combat infectious diseases. Specifically, preventing these pathogens from manipulating this crucial cellular pathway could lead to their eventual elimination.

Targeting pathogen-mediated autophagy interference is a promising avenue for therapeutic intervention. One approach is to develop drugs that restore normal autophagy function, such as autophagy inducers that promote the formation of autophagosomes or autophagy enhancers that facilitate the fusion of autophagosomes with lysosomes. These drugs could help clear pathogens from infected cells and reduce cellular stress and inflammation. Another approach is to develop drugs that specifically target pathogen proteins involved in autophagy interference. By blocking the interaction of these proteins with autophagy regulators, it may be possible to disrupt pathogen replication and dissemination. These targeted therapies could offer a more precise and effective way to combat infectious diseases, while minimizing the potential for off-target effects.

Ultimately, autophagy interference is a critical aspect of pathogen pathogenesis. By understanding the diverse mechanisms by which pathogens manipulate autophagy, we can develop new and improved strategies to combat infectious diseases and protect human health. This understanding can pave the way for novel therapeutic interventions that target pathogen-mediated autophagy interference, ultimately helping to restore cellular homeostasis and enhance the host's ability to fight infection. Further research in this area is crucial for developing effective therapies against a wide range of infectious agents, including viruses, bacteria, and parasites. As we continue to unravel the complexities of autophagy and its interactions with pathogens, we can expect to see the development of innovative strategies to combat infectious diseases.

4.3 Golgi Network Disruption

Within the intricate labyrinth of cellular machinery, the Golgi network stands as a central processing and packaging hub. This organelle, a stack of flattened, membrane-bound sacs called cisternae, diligently modifies, sorts, and ships proteins and lipids to their final destinations within and outside the cell. However, this crucial function is often targeted and disrupted by cunning infectious agents, particularly viruses and certain bacteria, to facilitate their own replication and spread. These pathogens have evolved sophisticated strategies to hijack the Golgi, turning it from a cellular asset into a tool for their own survival, thus the disruption of its network.

The effects of Golgi network disruption by infectious agents are far-reaching, with consequences extending to both host cell function and pathogen replication. One of the most significant impacts is the impairment of protein glycosylation, the process by which sugars are added to proteins. This modification is essential for proper protein folding, stability, and trafficking. Many viral glycoproteins, for instance, require glycosylation for their assembly and infectivity, or they can be secreted in the environment, not allowing a proper cellular interaction. By disrupting the Golgi, pathogens can interfere with the glycosylation of host cell proteins, leading to cellular dysfunction. Conversely, they can also manipulate glycosylation to their own advantage, ensuring the proper folding and function of their own viral proteins. Furthermore, this disruption can lead to the accumulation of unfolded or misfolded proteins within the endoplasmic reticulum (ER), triggering the unfolded protein response (UPR), a cellular stress pathway that can have both protective and detrimental effects.

Moreover, the Golgi network is critical for the trafficking of proteins and lipids to various cellular compartments, including the plasma membrane, lysosomes, and secretory vesicles. Pathogens can disrupt this trafficking machinery to redirect cellular resources to their replication sites. For example, some viruses induce the formation of viral replication factories near the Golgi, effectively commandeering the organelle to facilitate viral assembly and budding. This redirection of resources can compromise the host cell's ability to carry out its normal functions, weakening its defenses and increasing its susceptibility to infection. Moreover, disruption of Golgi-mediated trafficking can also interfere with the secretion of cytokines and other immune signaling molecules, impairing the host's ability to mount an effective immune response.

Viral infection often leads to a fragmented and disorganized Golgi apparatus, a consequence of the virus's direct or indirect effects on the structural and functional components of the organelle. Some viruses, such as certain influenza strains, encode proteins that directly interact with Golgi proteins, disrupting their normal function. These viral proteins may interfere with the assembly of the Golgi stack, block the transport of proteins through the Golgi, or induce the disassembly of the organelle altogether. Other viruses, such as some coronaviruses, induce changes in lipid metabolism that can affect the structure and function of the Golgi membranes. The fragmented Golgi can then become a hub for viral replication and assembly, providing a protected environment for the virus to multiply.

Beyond viruses, certain bacteria also target the Golgi network to promote their intracellular survival and spread. Some bacteria secrete toxins that directly disrupt Golgi function, while others manipulate host cell signaling pathways to alter Golgi structure and trafficking. For example, some bacteria inject effector proteins into host cells that interfere with the recruitment of coat proteins to the Golgi membrane, disrupting protein trafficking. Other bacteria manipulate host cell signaling pathways, such as the PI3K/Akt pathway, to promote the formation of bacterial replication vacuoles near the Golgi, creating a niche for bacterial replication. The consequence for infected cells can be severe, with consequences that range from cell dysfunction to programmed cell death, depending on the bacterial species and the severity of the disruption.

Considering the critical role of the Golgi network in cellular function and pathogen replication, targeting Golgi disruption represents a promising avenue for therapeutic intervention. Strategies aimed at restoring Golgi function or preventing pathogen-induced Golgi disruption could potentially limit pathogen replication and reduce the severity of infection. One approach involves developing drugs that specifically target viral or bacterial proteins that interact with the Golgi, preventing them from disrupting the organelle's function. Another approach involves targeting host cell signaling pathways that are manipulated by pathogens to alter Golgi structure and trafficking, restoring normal Golgi function and preventing pathogen replication.

In fact, researchers are actively exploring a variety of therapeutic strategies to target Golgi network disruption. Some are focusing on developing small molecules that can inhibit the activity of viral or bacterial proteins that disrupt Golgi function. Others are investigating the potential of using RNA interference (RNAi) to silence the expression of these proteins. Still others are exploring the use of immunomodulatory therapies to restore normal Golgi function and enhance the host's immune response. While many of these strategies are still in the early stages of development, they hold great promise for improving our ability to combat infectious diseases.

The Golgi network's vulnerability to pathogen-mediated disruption highlights the importance of understanding the intricate interplay between pathogens and host cells at the subcellular level. By further elucidating the mechanisms by which pathogens manipulate the Golgi, we can develop more effective strategies to prevent and treat infectious diseases. Such insights not only inform the development of novel therapeutic interventions but also deepen our understanding of fundamental cellular processes and the dynamic interactions between pathogens and their hosts. The future of infectious disease control may well lie in our ability to target and manipulate these intricate interactions within the cellular realm.

5 Chapter 5: Immune Evasion Tactics

Pathogens, masters of survival, have evolved a sophisticated arsenal of strategies to evade the relentless assault of the host's immune system. These tactics, honed over millennia of co-evolution, allow them to persist, replicate, and ultimately, cause disease. Understanding these evasive maneuvers is crucial for developing effective vaccines and therapeutic interventions that can outsmart these cunning invaders. It's a constant arms race, and we must stay ahead to protect human health.

Antigenic variation stands as a cornerstone of immune evasion, particularly for viruses and certain bacteria. This involves altering surface antigens, the very molecules that the immune system recognizes and targets. Imagine trying to hit a constantly moving target; that's the challenge antigenic variation presents to our immune defenses. Viruses like influenza, for example, employ antigenic drift and antigenic shift. Antigenic drift involves minor, gradual mutations in the viral genes encoding surface proteins like hemagglutinin (HA) and neuraminidase (NA). These subtle changes accumulate over time, leading to new viral strains that are no longer effectively recognized by antibodies generated against previous strains. This is why we need annual flu vaccines, each tailored to the predicted circulating strains. Antigenic shift, on the other hand, is a more dramatic event, involving the reassortment of entire gene segments between different viral strains. This can result in the sudden emergence of completely novel viruses, against which the population has little or no pre-existing immunity, potentially triggering pandemics. HIV, the virus that causes AIDS, also relies heavily on antigenic variation. Its high mutation rate, coupled with its error-prone reverse transcriptase enzyme, leads to a constant stream of viral variants. This makes it extremely difficult for the immune system to clear the infection, and it also poses a significant challenge for vaccine development. Bacteria, too, can employ antigenic variation. Neisseria gonorrhoeae, the causative agent of gonorrhea, uses phase variation to alter the expression of its surface pili, which are involved in attachment to host cells. By switching pili expression on and off, the bacteria can evade antibody-mediated clearance. Similarly, Borrelia burgdorferi, the bacterium responsible for Lyme disease, undergoes antigenic variation of its outer surface protein VlsE, allowing it to persist in the host for extended periods. I saw a particularly compelling study demonstrating how even subtle glycosylation changes on bacterial surface antigens could dramatically impact antibody binding affinity, highlighting the exquisite sensitivity of the immune system to even minor structural alterations.

The complement system is a critical component of the innate immune response, acting as a rapid and potent defense against invading pathogens. However, many pathogens have evolved mechanisms to inhibit complement activation, effectively disarming this crucial arm of the immune system. Some bacteria produce molecules that directly interfere with the complement cascade. For example, Streptococcus pneumoniae produces a capsule composed of polysaccharide that inhibits the deposition of C3b, a key opsonin that facilitates phagocytosis. Similarly, Staphylococcus aureus expresses the staphylococcal complement inhibitor (SCIN), which binds to C3 convertase, preventing its activation and subsequent complement cascade amplification. Viruses can also target the complement system. Some viruses encode proteins that mimic or bind to complement regulatory proteins, effectively hijacking the host's own mechanisms for controlling complement activation. For instance, vaccinia virus, the virus used in the smallpox vaccine, produces the vaccinia virus complement control protein (VCP), which is homologous to human complement regulatory proteins like C4bp. VCP binds to C3b and C4b, preventing their activation and inhibiting the complement cascade. HIV also employs several strategies to evade complement. Viral particles incorporate host cell complement regulatory proteins like CD55 (DAF) and CD59 into their envelope, protecting them from complement-mediated lysis. Furthermore, HIV-infected cells can also upregulate the expression of these complement regulatory proteins, providing additional protection against complement attack. I recall a fascinating experiment where researchers showed that blocking CD59 on HIV-infected cells significantly increased their susceptibility to complement-mediated lysis, underscoring the importance of this evasion mechanism. These complement evasion strategies highlight the intricate ways in which pathogens can subvert the host's immune defenses, allowing them to persist and cause disease. Understanding these mechanisms is crucial for developing therapies that can restore complement function and enhance pathogen clearance.

Cytokine storms, characterized by excessive and dysregulated production of pro-inflammatory cytokines, can lead to severe tissue damage and even death. While the immune system uses cytokines to orchestrate the immune response, pathogens can manipulate this delicate balance to their advantage. Some pathogens induce excessive cytokine production, leading to a damaging cytokine storm. For example, highly pathogenic influenza viruses, such as the H5N1 avian influenza virus, can trigger a massive release of cytokines, including TNF-, IL-1, and IL-6. This "cytokine storm" contributes to acute respiratory distress syndrome (ARDS) and multi-organ failure, often resulting in fatal outcomes. Similarly, Staphylococcus aureus, during toxic shock syndrome, releases superantigens that activate a large proportion of T cells, leading to a massive cytokine release. This uncontrolled cytokine storm can cause fever, hypotension, and shock. On the other hand, some pathogens actively suppress cytokine production, weakening the host's immune response. For instance, measles virus inhibits the production of interferon (IFN), a critical cytokine for antiviral defense. This suppression of IFN allows the virus to replicate more efficiently and spread to other cells. HIV also suppresses cytokine production through various mechanisms. The virus infects and depletes CD4+ T cells, which are essential for producing cytokines that activate other immune cells. Furthermore, HIV can induce the production of immunosuppressive cytokines like IL-10, which dampen the immune response and promote viral persistence. I remember attending a conference where a researcher presented compelling data showing how certain viral proteins directly interact with cellular signaling pathways to inhibit cytokine gene expression, highlighting the complexity of these regulatory mechanisms. Therefore, it becomes clear that this careful modulation and regulation are crucial for the virus to maintain itself. The strategies pathogens employ to modulate cytokine production are diverse and complex, highlighting the intricate interplay between the pathogen and the host immune system. Understanding these mechanisms is essential for developing therapies that can either dampen excessive cytokine production in the case of cytokine storms or boost cytokine production in the case of immune suppression, ultimately restoring immune homeostasis and improving patient outcomes. The balance of these modulations is what separates the successful pathogens from the vulnerable ones.

5.1 Antigenic Variation

Antigenic variation is a cunning and remarkably effective strategy employed by numerous infectious agents to outwit the host's immune system. It's a dynamic game of molecular hide-and-seek, where pathogens alter their surface antigens, the very molecules that the immune system uses to recognize and target them. This constant reshaping of their identity allows these organisms to evade existing immunity, leading to persistent infections and posing significant challenges for vaccine development. Understanding the intricacies of antigenic variation is therefore crucial for devising effective strategies to combat infectious diseases.

One of the most well-studied examples of antigenic variation is seen in influenza viruses. These viruses, notorious for causing seasonal epidemics, undergo two primary mechanisms of antigenic change: antigenic drift and antigenic shift. Antigenic drift refers to the accumulation of small point mutations in the genes encoding the viral surface glycoproteins, hemagglutinin (HA) and neuraminidase (NA). These mutations, driven by the error-prone nature of the viral RNA polymerase, gradually alter the structure of HA and NA, diminishing the binding affinity of pre-existing antibodies. This means that individuals who were previously immune to a particular strain of influenza may become susceptible to a slightly mutated version, leading to repeated outbreaks. Antigenic shift, on the other hand, is a more dramatic and less frequent event. It involves the reassortment of entire gene segments between different influenza viruses, typically occurring when two different strains infect the same host cell. This can result in the sudden emergence of a completely novel influenza virus with a drastically different HA and/or NA protein, against which the human population has little to no pre-existing immunity. Antigenic shift is responsible for the devastating influenza pandemics that have occurred throughout history.

Beyond influenza, a diverse range of pathogens utilize antigenic variation to their advantage. The African trypanosomes, which cause sleeping sickness, employ a particularly sophisticated strategy known as variant surface glycoprotein (VSG) switching. These parasites are covered in a dense coat of VSG molecules, which act as a protective shield against the host's immune system. However, the trypanosome genome contains hundreds of different VSG genes, only one of which is expressed at any given time. Through a process of gene rearrangement, the parasite can switch from expressing one VSG to another, thereby presenting a new antigenic face to the immune system. This constant switching allows the trypanosomes to persist in the host bloodstream for extended periods, evading antibody-mediated clearance. Similarly, Plasmodium falciparum, the causative agent of malaria, expresses a family of variant surface antigens called PfEMP1 on the surface of infected red blood cells. PfEMP1 mediates the adhesion of infected red blood cells to the lining of blood vessels, preventing their clearance by the spleen. The parasite possesses a vast repertoire of PfEMP1 genes, which it can switch between to evade antibody responses and maintain chronic infection.

The mechanisms underlying antigenic variation are equally diverse. Some pathogens, like influenza, rely on mutation and reassortment. Others, like trypanosomes, employ gene switching. Still others, such as Neisseria gonorrhoeae, the bacterium responsible for gonorrhea, utilize DNA recombination to generate antigenic diversity in their pilin proteins, which are involved in attachment to host cells. These pilin proteins undergo frequent changes in their amino acid sequence due to recombination events, making it difficult for the immune system to generate long-lasting immunity. Furthermore, some pathogens, like HIV, combine multiple strategies, employing both high mutation rates and glycosylation patterns to shield their surface antigens from antibody recognition.

Understanding the mechanisms by which pathogens achieve antigenic variation is critical for developing effective vaccines and therapies. Traditional vaccine approaches, which rely on inducing antibody responses against specific antigens, can be rendered ineffective by antigenic variation. Therefore, researchers are exploring alternative strategies that can overcome this challenge. One approach is to develop broadly neutralizing antibodies that target conserved epitopes, regions of the antigen that are less prone to mutation. Another strategy is to develop vaccines that elicit cellular immune responses, such as T cell responses, which can recognize and kill infected cells regardless of antigenic variation. Furthermore, researchers are investigating the possibility of targeting the mechanisms of antigenic variation itself, for example, by inhibiting the enzymes involved in gene switching or recombination.

The implications of antigenic variation extend beyond vaccine development. Diagnostic tests that rely on detecting specific antigens can also be affected by antigenic variation, leading to false-negative results. Moreover, the ability of pathogens to evade the immune system through antigenic variation can contribute to the development of chronic infections and the emergence of drug resistance. Therefore, a comprehensive understanding of antigenic variation is essential for addressing the challenges posed by emerging and re-emerging infectious diseases. As we continue to face the threat of novel pathogens and the spread of existing ones, the study of antigenic variation will remain a crucial area of research. By unraveling the secrets of this evasive strategy, we can develop more effective tools to protect ourselves against the ever-evolving world of infectious agents. It requires innovative thinking and a multidisciplinary approach, bringing together expertise from immunology, virology, bacteriology, and molecular biology. This collaborative effort is crucial for staying one step ahead in the ongoing arms race between pathogens and the host immune system.

5.2 Complement Inhibition

The complement system, a crucial arm of the innate immune system, acts as a first responder, rapidly identifying and eliminating pathogens. Think of it as a cascading series of protein activations, where each step amplifies the signal, leading to a potent attack on invaders.

However, this powerful system, if unchecked, can also damage host tissues. Thus, pathogens have evolved ingenious strategies to inhibit complement activation, allowing them to evade immune destruction and establish infection. This chapter will explore these cunning tactics employed by viruses and bacteria, focusing on the mechanisms and consequences of complement inhibition. We'll look at specific examples and highlight the significance of these strategies in the context of infectious disease.
The classical pathway, triggered by antibody-antigen complexes, is a prime target for pathogens. Certain bacteria produce surface proteins that directly bind to antibodies, preventing them from effectively activating the C1 complex, the initiator of the classical pathway. Imagine a bacterial cell cloaking itself in a disguise that renders it invisible to the classical pathway's surveillance system. Some pathogens even go a step further, secreting proteases that degrade complement components like C1q, directly disrupting the pathway's initiation. This enzymatic degradation acts as a molecular sabotage, disabling the classical pathway before it can even get started. Viruses, too, employ similar strategies; some encode proteins that mimic complement control proteins, effectively disrupting the assembly of the C1 complex. The consequences

of this inhibition are significant: reduced opsonization (marking pathogens for phagocytosis), diminished inflammation, and impaired pathogen clearance, all contributing to enhanced survival of the infectious agent.

Then we have the alternative pathway, which provides continuous surveillance for pathogens. This pathway is initiated by spontaneous hydrolysis of C3, a key complement component. Normally, regulatory proteins like Factor H and Factor I quickly inactivate the spontaneously activated C3b, preventing uncontrolled amplification. However, some pathogens produce surface molecules that bind to Factor H, recruiting it to their surface. This seemingly innocuous act turns Factor H into a shield, protecting the pathogen from complement-mediated damage. Other pathogens express molecules that accelerate the decay of the C3 convertase, the enzyme responsible for amplifying the alternative pathway. By destabilizing this enzyme, they effectively dampen the entire pathway's response. A fascinating example is found in certain strains of bacteria that produce a capsule rich in sialic acid. Sialic acid binds Factor H, promoting its association with the bacterial surface and inhibiting complement activation. It's a clever disguise, allowing the bacteria to blend in with the host's own cells, which are also decorated with sialic acid.

Moreover, the lectin pathway, activated by the recognition of microbial carbohydrates, presents another avenue for pathogens to subvert complement. Mannose-binding lectin (MBL) and ficolins recognize specific sugar patterns on the surface of bacteria, fungi, and viruses, initiating a cascade similar to the classical pathway. Pathogens can interfere with this pathway by producing glycans that mask their own mannose-rich surfaces, preventing MBL from binding. Think of it as a game of hide-and-seek, where the pathogen cleverly conceals its identifying features to avoid detection. Some viruses go even further, encoding proteins that bind to MBL, preventing it from activating the downstream complement components. This interaction acts as a molecular decoy, diverting MBL away from its intended target and preventing the initiation of the lectin pathway. The implications of these inhibitory strategies are profound, allowing pathogens to evade complement-mediated opsonization, inflammation, and direct lysis.

One should know that the membrane attack complex (MAC), the end result of all three complement pathways, forms pores in the pathogen's membrane, leading to lysis. This powerful weapon is a major threat to bacteria and enveloped viruses. To counter this threat, many pathogens have evolved strategies to inhibit MAC formation. Some bacteria produce surface molecules that prevent the insertion of C5b-9, the components of the MAC, into their membrane. Others express proteases that degrade the MAC components, disrupting its assembly. Even viruses can encode proteins that interfere with MAC formation, preventing it from effectively puncturing the viral envelope. These inhibitory strategies are crucial for pathogens to survive complement attack and establish a successful infection.

Furthermore, understanding the mechanisms of complement inhibition is vital for developing novel therapeutic strategies. Blocking these inhibitory pathways could restore complement activity and enhance pathogen clearance. For example, researchers are exploring the use of small molecule inhibitors that target the pathogen's complement-inhibitory proteins, effectively disabling their protective shields. Another approach involves developing antibodies that neutralize these inhibitory molecules, allowing the complement system to function unimpeded. These therapeutic interventions hold promise for combating infectious diseases by bolstering the host's natural defenses.

As a closing, let's consider some specific examples to illustrate the impact of complement inhibition. Streptococcus pneumoniae, a common cause of pneumonia and meningitis, produces a capsule that inhibits complement activation. This capsule prevents C3b deposition on the bacterial surface, reducing opsonization and phagocytosis. Neisseria meningitidis, the causative agent of meningococcal meningitis, expresses a surface protein called factor H binding protein (fHbp) that recruits Factor H, inhibiting the alternative pathway. HIV-1 incorporates host complement regulatory proteins, such as CD59, into its viral envelope, protecting it from complement-mediated lysis. These examples highlight the diverse and sophisticated strategies pathogens employ to evade complement. By understanding these strategies, we can develop targeted therapies to overcome complement inhibition and improve the treatment of infectious diseases. The ongoing battle between pathogens and the complement system is a testament to the power of natural selection, driving the evolution of ever more cunning evasion tactics and prompting us to develop innovative countermeasures.

5.3 Cytokine Storm Modulation

The uncontrolled surge of cytokines, often referred to as a cytokine storm, represents a paradoxical outcome of the host's defense mechanisms against invading pathogens. While cytokines are crucial signaling molecules that orchestrate immune responses, their excessive and dysregulated production can lead to systemic inflammation, tissue damage, and potentially fatal outcomes. Understanding how pathogens manipulate cytokine production and signaling pathways is paramount for developing effective therapeutic strategies to mitigate the detrimental effects of cytokine storms. Several viruses have mastered methods to amplify or suppress cytokine synthesis, including interferon, interleukins, TNF, and chemokines.

Pathogens employ diverse strategies to modulate the host's cytokine response, often tailoring their tactics to promote their own survival and replication. One common approach is to directly stimulate the excessive production of pro-inflammatory cytokines. For instance, certain viruses and bacteria can trigger the activation of pattern recognition receptors (PRRs), such as Toll-like receptors (TLRs), on immune cells. This activation initiates signaling cascades that lead to the upregulation of genes encoding pro-inflammatory cytokines like interleukin-1 (IL-1), interleukin-6 (IL-6), and tumor necrosis factor- (TNF-). The excessive release of these cytokines can overwhelm the host's regulatory mechanisms, resulting in a systemic inflammatory response syndrome (SIRS) and, in severe cases, acute respiratory distress syndrome (ARDS) or multiple organ dysfunction syndrome (MODS). Furthermore, some pathogens produce superantigens, toxins that bypass normal antigen processing and directly stimulate T cells. This non-specific T cell activation leads to the massive release of cytokines, contributing to the cytokine storm.

Conversely, pathogens can also employ strategies to suppress the host's cytokine response, particularly those cytokines involved in antiviral or antibacterial defense. Some viruses encode proteins that interfere with the signaling pathways downstream of PRRs, effectively blocking the production of interferon (IFN), a critical cytokine for antiviral immunity. By suppressing IFN production, these viruses can evade the host's initial antiviral defenses and establish a more persistent infection. Other pathogens produce decoy receptors that bind to cytokines, preventing them from interacting with their cognate receptors on immune cells and dampening the inflammatory response. This immunosuppressive strategy can promote pathogen survival and replication, but it can also leave the host vulnerable to secondary infections.

Targeting cytokine storm modulation represents a crucial avenue for therapeutic intervention in severe infectious diseases. Several strategies are currently being explored and implemented to mitigate the detrimental effects of excessive cytokine production. One approach involves the use of broad-spectrum immunosuppressants, such as corticosteroids, to dampen the overall inflammatory response. While corticosteroids can be effective in reducing inflammation, they also carry the risk of suppressing the host's immune system, potentially increasing susceptibility to secondary infections. More targeted therapies that specifically block the action of key pro-inflammatory cytokines are also being developed. For example, monoclonal antibodies that neutralize IL-6 or TNF-have shown promise in clinical trials for treating cytokine storms associated with certain infections. These antibodies can selectively inhibit the signaling pathways mediated by these cytokines, reducing inflammation without causing widespread immunosuppression.

Another therapeutic approach focuses on modulating the signaling pathways that regulate cytokine production. Small molecule inhibitors that target kinases involved in the activation of inflammatory signaling pathways are being investigated as potential therapeutic agents. These inhibitors can selectively block the production of pro-inflammatory cytokines by interfering with the signaling cascades triggered by PRR activation. Furthermore, therapies that enhance the production of anti-inflammatory cytokines, such as IL-10, are also being explored. IL-10 can suppress the production of pro-inflammatory cytokines and promote the resolution of inflammation, helping to restore immune homeostasis.

In addition to targeting cytokine production and signaling, therapeutic strategies that aim to remove excess cytokines from the circulation are also being developed. Cytokine adsorption devices, which filter blood to remove specific cytokines, have shown promise in clinical settings for treating cytokine storms associated with sepsis and other inflammatory conditions. These devices can rapidly reduce cytokine levels in the blood, potentially mitigating the systemic inflammatory response.

As an expert I can affirm that understanding the complex interplay between pathogens and the host's cytokine response is essential for developing effective therapeutic strategies to combat infectious diseases. Pathogens have evolved sophisticated mechanisms to manipulate cytokine production and signaling, and therapeutic interventions must be tailored to address the specific pathogenic mechanisms involved. By targeting key pro-inflammatory cytokines, modulating signaling pathways, and removing excess cytokines from the circulation, it is possible to mitigate the detrimental effects of cytokine storms and improve outcomes in patients with severe infections. The road towards mastering the modulation of the cytokine storm is long, and the goal is far but very achievable.

6 Chapter 6: Host Cell Signaling Modulation

Pathogens, in their relentless pursuit of replication, have evolved intricate mechanisms to manipulate host cell signaling pathways, effectively turning cellular machinery to their own advantage. One of the most crucial pathways targeted is the NF-B (Nuclear Factor kappa B) pathway. This pathway is a central regulator of inflammation, immunity, and cell survival, playing a vital role in the host's response to infection. Viruses and bacteria alike have developed strategies to either activate or inhibit NF-B signaling, depending on their needs at different stages of infection. Some viruses, for example, initially activate NF-B to promote their own replication by inducing the expression of viral genes or suppressing antiviral responses. However, at later stages, they may inhibit NF-B to prevent the host from mounting an effective immune response, or to promote cell survival and establish persistence. Bacteria, on the other hand, may activate NF-B to induce inflammation, which can damage host tissues and facilitate their spread, or they may inhibit NF-B to evade immune detection and clearance. The specific mechanisms of NF-B modulation vary depending on the pathogen and the host cell type, but they often involve the manipulation of upstream kinases, ubiquitin ligases, or transcriptional regulators.

The interferon (IFN) response is another critical arm of the host's antiviral defense. IFNs are a family of cytokines that induce the expression of hundreds of genes involved in antiviral immunity, including pattern recognition receptors, antiviral enzymes, and chemokines. To counteract this potent defense, many viruses have evolved strategies to block the IFN response at various steps. Some viruses interfere with the production of IFNs by inhibiting the activation of transcription factors such as IRF3 or NF-B, which are required for IFN gene expression. Others target the IFN receptors on the cell surface, preventing IFN signaling from occurring. Still others inhibit the activity of downstream antiviral enzymes, such as RNase L or PKR, which are activated by IFN signaling. These mechanisms allow viruses to replicate more efficiently in the presence of

IFNs, increasing their virulence and transmissibility. Effective evasion of the IFN response is often a key determinant of viral pathogenesis.

The Mitogen-Activated Protein Kinase (MAPK) signaling cascades, comprising ERK, JNK, and p38 pathways, are vital for translating extracellular stimuli into intracellular responses, influencing processes like cell growth, differentiation, and apoptosis. Pathogens adeptly manipulate these pathways to foster their survival and propagation. Viruses, for instance, can activate the ERK pathway to promote cell proliferation, creating a conducive environment for viral replication. Conversely, they might induce the JNK pathway to trigger apoptosis in immune cells, suppressing the host's defense mechanisms. Bacteria, similarly, can exploit MAPK pathways to enhance their invasion and colonization. Some bacterial toxins activate p38 MAPK, leading to the production of pro-inflammatory cytokines that damage host tissues, while others inhibit MAPK signaling to evade immune surveillance. Disruption of MAPK pathways allows pathogens to orchestrate cellular responses in their favor, ultimately promoting their survival and dissemination.

Apoptosis, or programmed cell death, is a crucial cellular process that eliminates infected or damaged cells, preventing the spread of pathogens. However, many pathogens have evolved strategies to regulate apoptosis, either by inducing it to facilitate their release or by inhibiting it to prolong the lifespan of infected cells. Viruses, for instance, often induce apoptosis in the late stages of infection to release viral particles and spread to new cells. They may also inhibit apoptosis in the early stages of infection to maintain a permissive environment for viral replication. Bacteria, on the other hand, may induce apoptosis in immune cells to suppress the host's immune response or inhibit apoptosis in infected epithelial cells to prolong their survival and promote bacterial colonization. The regulation of apoptosis is a complex interplay between host and pathogen, with the outcome often determining the fate of the infection. This intricate balance is finely tuned, and pathogens have evolved multiple strategies to manipulate it for their benefit.

The Phosphatidylinositol 3-Kinase (PI3K)/Akt pathway is a central regulator of cell growth, survival, and metabolism, making it a prime target for pathogens. Viruses, for example, can activate the PI3K/Akt pathway to promote cell survival and create a more favorable environment for viral replication. Activation of Akt can also inhibit apoptosis, prolonging the lifespan of infected cells. Furthermore, the PI3K/Akt pathway can regulate glucose metabolism, providing pathogens with the energy and building blocks they need to replicate. Bacteria can also manipulate the PI3K/Akt pathway to promote their survival and spread. Some bacteria secrete toxins that activate the PI3K/Akt pathway, leading to increased cell survival and proliferation. Others inhibit the pathway to suppress the host's immune response. Understanding how pathogens influence the PI3K/Akt pathway is crucial for developing targeted therapies that can disrupt their replication and spread. Further research into these complex interactions promises to unveil novel therapeutic avenues for combating infectious diseases.

6.1 NF-B Pathway Control

Consider the NF-B pathway, a central regulator of immune responses and inflammation; it acts as a critical control point that infectious disease agents frequently target for manipulation, understanding how these agents exert this control is paramount to designing effective therapeutic interventions. These pathways, when dysregulated, can lead to devastating consequences, like cytokine storms or chronic inflammatory conditions.

At the heart of the NF-B pathway lies a family of transcription factors that, when activated, translocate to the nucleus and induce the expression of genes involved in immune cell activation, cytokine production, and cell survival, many pathogens have evolved sophisticated strategies to either activate or inhibit this pathway, depending on their specific needs for survival and replication within the host. Activation of NF-B typically occurs through a cascade of events triggered by pattern recognition receptors (PRRs) that recognize pathogen-associated molecular patterns (PAMPs). For example, viral RNA can be recognized by toll-like receptors (TLRs) located on endosomal membranes, leading to the recruitment of adaptor proteins, activation of kinases, and ultimately, the phosphorylation and degradation of IB proteins, which normally sequester NF-B in the cytoplasm. Once freed from IB, NF-B dimers translocate to the nucleus and bind to specific DNA sequences in the promoter regions of target genes. This seemingly simple pathway is actually a complex network involving numerous regulatory proteins and feedback loops, providing multiple points of intervention for pathogens.

Many viruses, for instance, actively promote NF-B activation early in infection to create a cellular environment that favors their replication; this initial activation can enhance the production of antiviral cytokines and chemokines, which can help to control the spread of the infection. However, unchecked NF-B activation can also lead to excessive inflammation and tissue damage. Therefore, some viruses also encode proteins that inhibit NF-B activation at later stages of infection to suppress the host's immune response and establish persistent infection. These viral inhibitors can target various steps in the NF-B pathway, such as blocking the activation of upstream kinases, interfering with the degradation of IB proteins, or preventing the binding of NF-B to DNA. The strategies employed by bacteria are similarly diverse. Some bacteria, like Salmonella, inject effector proteins into host cells that directly activate NF-B, leading to the production of proinflammatory cytokines that contribute to the pathogenesis of the infection. Conversely, other bacteria, such as Yersinia, inject effector proteins that inhibit NF-B activation, suppressing the host's immune response and allowing the bacteria to proliferate unchecked.

Moreover, some infectious agents employ indirect mechanisms to modulate NF-B signaling. For instance, certain viruses can induce the production of cellular microRNAs that target components of the NF-B pathway, leading to either activation or inhibition of the pathway depending on the specific microRNA and its target. Understanding these intricate mechanisms of NF-B modulation is essential for developing effective therapeutic strategies. Therapies that aim to block excessive NF-B activation could be beneficial in cases of cytokine storms or chronic inflammatory conditions, while therapies that promote NF-B activation could be useful in boosting the host's immune response to clear persistent infections. Several drugs that target the NF-B pathway are already in clinical use or in development. For example, corticosteroids are widely used to suppress inflammation by inhibiting the expression of NF-B target genes. Specific inhibitors of IB kinases (IKKs) are also being developed as potential therapies for inflammatory diseases and cancer.

Furthermore, novel therapeutic approaches are being explored that target pathogen-specific mechanisms of NF-B modulation, by specifically blocking the activity of viral or bacterial proteins that interfere with the pathway, it may be possible to restore normal immune function and control the infection without causing widespread immunosuppression. In addition to drug-based therapies, other strategies are being investigated to modulate NF-B signaling, gene therapy approaches that deliver specific inhibitors of the NF-B pathway to target cells, or, conversely,

gene therapy approaches that enhance the expression of NF-B activators in immunocompromised individuals. The future of infectious disease therapeutics lies in our ability to precisely target and modulate host cell signaling pathways, such as NF-B, to restore immune homeostasis and control the infection. By gaining a deeper understanding of the molecular mechanisms by which infectious agents manipulate these pathways, we can develop more effective and targeted therapies that minimize off-target effects and maximize therapeutic efficacy.
The battle between host and pathogen is a constant tug-of-war, and understanding the intricacies of NF-B pathway control is crucial to tipping the balance in our favor. Furthermore, the understanding of NF-kB mechanisms may require a holistic approach to consider the impact on other signaling pathways that are essential in the signaling cascade.

6.2 Interferon Response Blockade

The interferon response is a cornerstone of cellular defense against viral infections, a rapid and potent mechanism that mobilizes the host's resources to suppress viral replication and alert neighboring cells. However, many viruses have evolved sophisticated countermeasures to block or subvert this crucial defense, allowing them to establish infection and spread within the host. The success of these viral evasion strategies underscores the importance of understanding the intricate mechanisms of interferon signaling and the specific ways in which viruses interfere with this pathway. This chapter will explore the key steps in the interferon response and delve into the diverse tactics employed by viruses to negate its effects, providing a deeper understanding of viral pathogenesis and informing the development of more effective antiviral therapies.

The interferon response begins with the recognition of viral components by cellular sensors, such as Toll-like receptors (TLRs) located in endosomes or RIG-I-like receptors (RLRs) in the cytoplasm. These receptors detect viral nucleic acids, triggering a cascade of intracellular signaling events that ultimately lead to the activation of transcription factors like IRF3 and NF-B. These transcription factors then translocate to the nucleus, where they bind to specific DNA sequences in the promoter regions of interferon genes, initiating the transcription of type I interferons (IFN-/). The newly synthesized interferon proteins are secreted from the cell and bind to the interferon-/ receptor (IFNAR) on the surface of both infected and neighboring cells. This binding activates the JAK-STAT signaling pathway, leading to the phosphorylation and activation of STAT proteins, which then translocate to the nucleus and induce the expression of hundreds of interferon-stimulated genes (ISGs). ISGs encode proteins with diverse antiviral functions, including enzymes that inhibit viral replication, proteins that promote apoptosis of infected cells, and factors that enhance the activity of the adaptive immune system. The interferon response is a complex and highly regulated process, involving multiple signaling pathways and feedback loops that ensure an appropriate and timely antiviral response.

Viruses have evolved a remarkable array of strategies to block the interferon response at various stages of the pathway. Some viruses directly interfere with the detection of viral components by cellular sensors. For example, certain viruses encode proteins that sequester or degrade viral nucleic acids, preventing them from activating TLRs or RLRs. Others express proteins that interfere with the signaling pathways downstream of these receptors, blocking the activation of IRF3 or NF-B. One common tactic is to target the adaptor proteins that mediate signaling between the receptors and downstream kinases. By disrupting these interactions, viruses can effectively shut down the initial stages of the interferon response.

A second major strategy employed by viruses is to interfere with the expression or activity of interferon itself. Some viruses encode proteins that inhibit the transcription of interferon genes, preventing the production of interferon protein. Others express proteins that directly bind to and neutralize interferon, preventing it from binding to its receptor. Still others produce proteins that promote the degradation of interferon mRNA, reducing the levels of interferon protein in the cell. By targeting interferon itself, viruses can effectively disable the entire interferon response.

Another important target for viral interference is the JAK-STAT signaling pathway, which is essential for the induction of ISG expression. Many viruses encode proteins that block the phosphorylation of STAT proteins, preventing their activation and translocation to the nucleus. Others express proteins that interfere with the binding of STAT proteins to DNA, preventing the transcription of ISGs. Some viruses even encode proteins that promote the degradation of STAT proteins, reducing their levels in the cell. By targeting the JAK-STAT pathway, viruses can effectively block the expression of hundreds of antiviral proteins.

Finally, viruses can also interfere with the function of specific ISGs. Some viruses encode proteins that directly inhibit the activity of antiviral enzymes, such as RNase L, which degrades viral RNA, or PKR, which inhibits protein synthesis. Others express proteins that counteract the effects of apoptosis-inducing ISGs, preventing infected cells from undergoing programmed cell death. By targeting specific ISGs, viruses can selectively disable key components of the antiviral response.

The specific mechanisms of interferon response blockade vary depending on the virus and the host cell type. Some viruses, like influenza virus, employ multiple strategies to inhibit the interferon response at different stages of the pathway. The NS1 protein of influenza virus, for example, can bind to and sequester viral RNA, inhibit the activation of IRF3, and block the expression of interferon genes. Other viruses, like hepatitis C virus, rely on a single dominant mechanism to suppress the interferon response. The NS3/4A protease of hepatitis C virus, for example, cleaves and inactivates the adaptor protein MAVS, which is essential for RLR signaling.

Understanding the mechanisms by which viruses block the interferon response is crucial for developing effective antiviral therapies. One approach is to design drugs that target viral proteins involved in interferon antagonism, restoring the host's ability to mount an effective antiviral response. Another approach is to develop interferon-based therapies that can overcome viral blockade mechanisms, such as using high doses of interferon or developing modified interferons that are resistant to viral inhibition. A deeper understanding of the interplay between viruses and the interferon response will pave the way for the development of novel and more effective strategies to combat viral infections. We now understand that we need to be able to adapt to such attacks.

6.3 MAPK Signaling Alteration

The intricate dance between pathogen and host often hinges on the manipulation of critical signaling cascades within the host cell. Among these, the Mitogen-Activated Protein Kinase (MAPK) pathways stand out as prime targets for infectious agents. These pathways, evolutionarily conserved, act as central communication hubs, relaying extracellular stimuli to the nucleus to orchestrate a variety of cellular processes, including cell growth, differentiation, inflammation, and apoptosis. A disruption in MAPK signaling can have profound consequences, tipping the cellular balance in favor of the pathogen, enabling its replication, dissemination, and evasion of host defenses.

Viruses, bacteria, fungi, and parasites have evolved sophisticated strategies to hijack MAPK pathways for their own survival. One common tactic involves the direct activation of specific MAPK kinases, leading to the upregulation of pro-survival genes and the suppression of apoptosis. For instance, certain viruses encode proteins that mimic host growth factors, triggering sustained MAPK activation and promoting cell proliferation, thereby creating a more permissive environment for viral replication. Other pathogens employ effector molecules that directly bind to and activate MAPK kinases, circumventing normal upstream signaling cues. This aberrant activation can lead to chronic inflammation, tissue damage, and even contribute to the development of cancers associated with persistent infections. What is interesting is that the pathogens are so evolved that they can manipulate the cells to proliferate only if necessary for their own needs, but not in a completely uncontrolled way.

Conversely, some pathogens employ the opposite strategy: inhibiting MAPK signaling to dampen the host's immune response. This can be achieved through the production of virulence factors that interfere with the activation of MAPK kinases or promote the dephosphorylation of activated MAPKs, effectively shutting down the pathway. By suppressing MAPK-dependent inflammatory responses, pathogens can evade detection by the immune system and establish persistent infections. The mechanisms by which different pathogens achieve this are diverse and often highly specific to the host cell type and the particular MAPK pathway involved. Consider, for example, how some bacteria inject effector proteins directly into host cells via specialized secretion systems. These effector proteins can directly target MAPK kinases, preventing their activation and blocking downstream signaling. Understanding the nuances of these inhibitory mechanisms is crucial for designing targeted therapies that can restore normal MAPK signaling and enhance the host's ability to combat infection.

Furthermore, the specific MAPK pathway targeted by a pathogen can vary depending on the stage of infection and the cellular process the pathogen seeks to manipulate. The three major MAPK pathways – ERK1/2, p38, and JNK – each play distinct roles in cellular signaling. The ERK1/2 pathway is typically associated with cell growth and proliferation, while the p38 and JNK pathways are primarily involved in stress responses and inflammation. A pathogen might initially activate the ERK1/2 pathway to promote its entry and replication, then switch to inhibiting the p38 or JNK pathway to suppress the ensuing inflammatory response. This dynamic modulation of MAPK signaling highlights the remarkable adaptability of pathogens and their ability to fine-tune their interactions with the host cell.

The consequences of MAPK signaling alteration extend beyond simple immune evasion or pro-survival signaling. Dysregulation of these pathways can disrupt a multitude of cellular processes, including cytokine production, cell cycle control, and angiogenesis. For example, aberrant activation of the p38 MAPK pathway can lead to excessive production of pro-inflammatory cytokines, contributing to the development of cytokine storms, a life-threatening complication of severe infections. Similarly, interference with MAPK-dependent cell cycle control can promote uncontrolled cell proliferation, increasing the risk of cancer development. Given the central role of MAPK pathways in regulating these diverse cellular functions, it is not surprising that their dysregulation can have such far-reaching consequences for host health.

Targeting MAPK signaling pathways represents a promising avenue for therapeutic intervention against infectious diseases. Several strategies are currently being explored, including the development of small-molecule inhibitors that specifically block the activity of MAPK kinases. These inhibitors can potentially restore normal MAPK signaling, enhance the host's immune response, and limit pathogen replication. However, the development of MAPK inhibitors for clinical use has been challenging due to the potential for off-target effects and the complex interplay between different MAPK pathways. A more targeted approach involves developing drugs that specifically interfere with the interaction between pathogen effector molecules and host MAPK kinases. This could selectively disrupt the pathogen's ability to manipulate MAPK signaling without affecting normal cellular functions. Moreover, understanding the specific mechanisms by which different pathogens alter MAPK signaling is crucial for developing tailored therapies that are most effective against particular infections.

In addition to direct targeting of MAPK kinases, alternative therapeutic strategies are also being investigated. These include approaches that aim to modulate upstream regulators of MAPK signaling or enhance the activity of MAPK phosphatases, which negatively regulate MAPK activity. Furthermore, immunomodulatory therapies that can restore normal immune function may also indirectly influence MAPK signaling, helping to restore cellular homeostasis and combat infection.

Finally, future research should focus on elucidating the intricate details of pathogen-host interactions at the level of MAPK signaling. This includes identifying novel pathogen effector molecules that target MAPK pathways, characterizing the specific mechanisms by which these effector molecules alter MAPK signaling, and understanding the consequences of MAPK dysregulation for host cell function and immune responses. By gaining a deeper understanding of these processes, we can develop more effective and targeted therapies to combat infectious diseases and improve human health.

6.4 Apoptosis Regulation

Apoptosis, or programmed cell death, serves as a critical defense mechanism against infectious agents, ensuring that compromised cells are eliminated before they can become viral or bacterial factories. The tightly regulated process is far from a simple on/off switch; instead, it's a complex signaling cascade that can be either triggered or suppressed by both the host and the invading pathogen. Understanding these intricate regulatory pathways is paramount in developing effective therapeutic strategies to combat infectious diseases.

The intrinsic pathway, triggered by cellular stress such as DNA damage or oxidative stress, is a key initiator of apoptosis. When a cell experiences irreparable damage, proteins like p53 are activated, leading to the transcription of pro-apoptotic genes like BAX and BAK. These proteins oligomerize on the mitochondrial outer membrane, forming pores that release cytochrome c into the cytoplasm. Cytochrome c then binds to Apaf-1, forming the apoptosome, which activates caspase-9, a crucial initiator caspase. The extrinsic pathway, on the other hand, is activated by external signals, such as the binding of death ligands like TNF- or FasL to their respective receptors on the cell surface. This interaction recruits adaptor proteins like FADD, forming the death-inducing signaling complex (DISC), which directly activates caspase-8, another initiator caspase. Both pathways converge on a common execution pathway, involving the activation of effector caspases like caspase-3, -6, and -7. These caspases cleave various cellular proteins, leading to the characteristic morphological changes associated with apoptosis, including cell shrinkage, DNA fragmentation, and the formation of apoptotic bodies, which are then engulfed by phagocytes. Infectious agents frequently manipulate these apoptotic pathways to promote their own survival and replication.

Some viruses encode proteins that directly inhibit caspase activation, preventing the cell from undergoing programmed cell death. For example, certain herpesviruses express proteins that mimic or inhibit caspase-8, blocking the extrinsic pathway. Adenoviruses, on the other hand, produce proteins that inhibit the function of pro-apoptotic proteins like BAX, preventing the intrinsic pathway from being activated. Bacteria can also interfere with apoptosis, often through the secretion of toxins that disrupt cellular signaling pathways. Some bacterial toxins, for instance, can activate anti-apoptotic proteins like Bcl-2, preventing cytochrome c release from the mitochondria. Others can directly inhibit caspase activity, effectively shutting down the apoptotic machinery. Conversely, some pathogens actively induce apoptosis to facilitate their spread or evade immune detection. Certain viruses, for example, induce apoptosis in immune cells, such as T cells, to suppress the host's immune response. Bacteria can also induce apoptosis in host cells to release nutrients or create an environment conducive to their replication.

The balance between pro-apoptotic and anti-apoptotic signals determines the fate of the infected cell. The Bcl-2 family of proteins plays a critical role in regulating this balance. This family includes both pro-apoptotic members like BAX, BAK, and BID, and anti-apoptotic members like Bcl-2, Bcl-xL, and MCL-1. The relative abundance of these proteins determines whether a cell will undergo apoptosis or survive. Anti-apoptotic proteins prevent the oligomerization of BAX and BAK, thereby preventing cytochrome c release. Pro-apoptotic proteins, on the other hand, can neutralize the anti-apoptotic effects of Bcl-2 and Bcl-xL, promoting cytochrome c release and apoptosis. Cellular signaling pathways, such as the PI3K/Akt pathway and the MAPK pathway, also play a critical role in regulating apoptosis. The PI3K/Akt pathway, for example, promotes cell survival by activating anti-apoptotic proteins like Bcl-2 and inhibiting pro-apoptotic proteins like BAD. The MAPK pathway can either promote or inhibit apoptosis, depending on the specific stimuli and cellular context. Understanding how pathogens manipulate apoptosis regulation is crucial for developing effective therapeutic strategies. One approach involves targeting the pathogen's anti-apoptotic mechanisms. For example, small molecule inhibitors that block the activity of viral or bacterial anti-apoptotic proteins can restore the host cell's ability to undergo apoptosis, thereby eliminating the pathogen. Another approach involves enhancing the host cell's pro-apoptotic signaling pathways. For instance, drugs that activate caspase-8 or caspase-9 can trigger apoptosis in infected cells, even in the presence of pathogen-encoded anti-apoptotic proteins. Immunotherapeutic strategies, such as adoptive T cell therapy, can also be used to target infected cells and induce apoptosis. By engineering T cells to express receptors that recognize pathogen-specific antigens, it's possible to specifically target infected cells for elimination. Furthermore, understanding the interplay between apoptosis and other cellular processes, such as autophagy and inflammation, is essential for developing comprehensive therapeutic strategies. Dysregulation of apoptosis can contribute to chronic inflammation and tissue damage, so therapies that restore normal apoptotic function may also have anti-inflammatory effects. Conversely, dysregulation of autophagy can impair the clearance of apoptotic cells, leading to the accumulation of cellular debris and further inflammation. Thus, therapies that target both apoptosis and autophagy may be particularly effective in treating infectious diseases.

6.5 PI3K/Akt Pathway Influence

The PI3K/Akt pathway stands as a central node in cellular signaling, orchestrating a multitude of processes vital for cell survival, growth, proliferation, metabolism, and motility. When an infectious agent enters the picture, it can dramatically alter the course of this pathway, influencing the host cell's fate in profound ways. A deep dive into how infectious disease agents, like viruses and bacteria, manipulate this pathway is critical for understanding disease pathogenesis and identifying potential therapeutic targets. The initial activation of the PI3K/Akt pathway typically begins with the stimulation of receptor tyrosine kinases (RTKs) or G protein-coupled receptors (GPCRs) by growth factors or other extracellular stimuli. Upon stimulation, phosphatidylinositol-3-kinase (PI3K) is recruited and activated. PI3K then phosphorylates phosphatidylinositol-4,5-bisphosphate (PIP2) to generate phosphatidylinositol-3,4,5-trisphosphate (PIP3). PIP3 acts as a docking site for pleckstrin homology (PH) domain-containing proteins, including Akt, also known as protein kinase B (PKB), and phosphoinositide-dependent kinase-1 (PDK1). Once recruited, Akt is phosphorylated by PDK1 at threonine 308 and by mammalian target of rapamycin complex 2 (mTORC2) at serine 473, leading to its full activation. Activated Akt then phosphorylates a plethora of downstream targets, thereby regulating a wide range of cellular processes. Given its central role, it's no surprise that numerous infectious agents have evolved strategies to either activate or inhibit this pathway to their advantage.

Viral manipulation of the PI3K/Akt pathway is diverse and often depends on the specific virus and host cell type. Some viruses, for example, activate the PI3K/Akt pathway to promote viral entry, replication, or survival of infected cells. By activating Akt, viruses can enhance glucose metabolism, providing the necessary energy and building blocks for viral replication. Moreover, Akt activation can inhibit apoptosis, preventing premature cell death and allowing the virus to complete its replication cycle. A virus might achieve this activation by directly interacting with PI3K or RTKs, mimicking growth factor signaling, or by encoding proteins that activate downstream targets of Akt. Conversely, other viruses might inhibit the PI3K/Akt pathway to suppress the host's immune response. Inhibition of Akt can lead to reduced production of pro-inflammatory cytokines, thereby evading immune detection and prolonging infection. This inhibition might be achieved by viral proteins that directly bind to and inactivate PI3K or Akt, or by interfering with upstream signaling events. The complex interplay between viruses and the PI3K/Akt pathway highlights the adaptability of these pathogens in manipulating host cell machinery for their own benefit.

Bacteria also employ a range of strategies to modulate

the PI3K/Akt pathway. Some bacteria activate the pathway to facilitate their entry into host cells or to promote intracellular survival. For instance, certain bacteria secrete effector proteins that directly activate Akt, leading to cytoskeletal rearrangements that promote bacterial uptake. Activation of Akt can also inhibit the host's innate immune response, suppressing the production of reactive oxygen species (ROS) and other antimicrobial compounds. Furthermore, some bacteria exploit the PI3K/Akt pathway to manipulate autophagy, a cellular process that degrades and recycles damaged or unwanted cellular components. By activating Akt, bacteria can inhibit autophagy, preventing their degradation and promoting their intracellular survival. On the other hand, some bacteria inhibit the PI3K/Akt pathway to disrupt host cell function or to facilitate their dissemination. Inhibition of Akt can lead to impaired cell migration, allowing bacteria to spread more easily throughout the host. Additionally, some bacteria produce toxins that directly target PI3K or Akt, leading to cell death or dysfunction. The manipulation of the PI3K/Akt pathway by bacteria is a crucial aspect of their pathogenesis, allowing them to colonize, survive, and cause disease.

Understanding the specific mechanisms by which infectious agents manipulate the PI3K/Akt pathway is crucial for developing targeted therapies. For example, if a virus activates the pathway to promote its replication, inhibitors of PI3K or Akt could be used to block viral replication and promote cell death. Conversely, if a bacterium inhibits the pathway to suppress the immune response, activators of PI3K or Akt could be used to boost the host's defenses and clear the infection. In addition to directly targeting PI3K or Akt, therapeutic strategies could also focus on modulating upstream or downstream components of the pathway. For instance, inhibitors of RTKs could prevent the initial activation of PI3K, while activators of downstream targets of Akt could restore normal cellular function. The development of effective therapies requires a detailed understanding of the specific signaling events that are disrupted by the infectious agent. By identifying the key points of intervention, researchers can design targeted drugs that effectively combat infection while minimizing side effects. This personalized approach to therapy holds great promise for the treatment of infectious diseases.

In conclusion, the PI3K/Akt pathway serves as a critical battleground in the host-pathogen interaction. Both viruses and bacteria have evolved sophisticated mechanisms to manipulate this pathway, either activating or inhibiting it to promote their own survival and replication. A thorough understanding of these mechanisms is essential for developing effective therapeutic strategies that can target the specific signaling events disrupted by infectious agents. As we continue to unravel the intricacies of the PI3K/Akt pathway and its interaction with various pathogens, we can pave the way for innovative therapies that will ultimately improve patient outcomes and combat the ever-evolving threat of infectious diseases.

7 Chapter 7: Therapeutic Intervention Avenues

The fight against infectious diseases hinges significantly on our ability to develop and deploy effective therapeutic interventions. These interventions can broadly be categorized into antiviral drug design, antibacterial strategies, and immunomodulatory approaches, each with its own set of challenges and opportunities. Understanding the molecular mechanisms of infection, as detailed in previous chapters, is paramount for rational drug design and the development of targeted therapies.

Antiviral drug design represents a cornerstone of our efforts to combat viral infections. A central strategy involves targeting specific stages of the viral replication cycle. For instance, drugs can be designed to inhibit viral entry by blocking the interaction between viral surface proteins and host cell receptors. Enfuvirtide, an HIV fusion inhibitor, serves as a prime example of this approach, preventing the virus from fusing with the host cell membrane. Other entry inhibitors are being developed to target different viruses and their specific receptor interactions. Another crucial target is the viral polymerase, the enzyme responsible for replicating the viral genome. Nucleoside analogs, such as acyclovir for herpesviruses and remdesivir for a range of RNA viruses, are incorporated into the growing viral DNA or RNA chain, causing premature termination and inhibiting replication. The key to success with these drugs lies in their selective toxicity, meaning they must effectively inhibit the viral polymerase without significantly affecting host cell polymerases. Protease inhibitors are another class of antiviral drugs that target viral enzymes. These drugs, widely used in HIV therapy, block the activity of viral proteases, enzymes that cleave viral polyproteins into functional proteins necessary for viral assembly. By inhibiting protease activity, these drugs prevent the production of infectious viral particles. Furthermore, research is focused on developing inhibitors of other viral enzymes, such as integrases and reverse transcriptases, to broaden the arsenal of available antiviral therapies. A challenge in antiviral drug design is the rapid evolution of viruses and the emergence of drug resistance. To combat this, researchers are exploring combination therapies, using multiple drugs that target different stages of the viral life cycle, thus reducing the likelihood of resistance development. Additionally, novel approaches are being investigated, such as targeting host cell factors that are essential for viral replication. This approach may offer a broader spectrum of activity and be less susceptible to resistance.

Antibacterial strategies are facing a crisis with the rise of antibiotic-resistant bacteria. The traditional approach of developing new antibiotics is becoming increasingly challenging, as bacteria are rapidly evolving resistance mechanisms. Consequently, researchers are exploring alternative strategies to combat bacterial infections. One promising approach is the development of novel antibacterial agents that target essential bacterial processes. For example, teixobactin, a recently discovered antibiotic, inhibits cell wall synthesis by binding to a highly conserved precursor molecule, making it less prone to resistance development. Another promising avenue is the development of antimicrobial peptides (AMPs), which are naturally occurring peptides with broad-spectrum antibacterial activity. AMPs can disrupt bacterial membranes, interfere with bacterial metabolism, or modulate the host immune response. They offer a potential alternative to traditional antibiotics, particularly for treating infections caused by multidrug-resistant bacteria. Phage therapy, which involves the use of bacteriophages (viruses that infect bacteria) to kill bacteria, is also gaining renewed interest. Phages are highly specific to their target bacteria and can effectively kill antibiotic-resistant strains. Phage therapy has shown promise in treating a variety of bacterial infections, including those caused by Staphylococcus aureus and Pseudomonas aeruginosa. Another area of focus is the development of inhibitors of bacterial virulence factors. Instead of killing bacteria directly, these drugs target the mechanisms that bacteria use to cause disease, such as toxins, adhesins, and biofilms. By inhibiting these virulence factors, the drugs can reduce the severity of infection and allow the host immune system to clear the bacteria. Furthermore, strategies to enhance the effectiveness of existing antibiotics are being explored, such as using antibiotic adjuvants that inhibit bacterial resistance mechanisms or improve antibiotic penetration into biofilms.

Immunomodulatory approaches represent a third category of therapeutic interventions that aim to harness the power of the host immune system to combat infectious diseases. These approaches can involve boosting the immune response to help clear the infection or suppressing the immune response to prevent excessive inflammation and tissue damage. One strategy is the use of cytokines, such as interferons and interleukins, to stimulate the immune system. Interferon-alpha, for example, is used to treat hepatitis C virus infection by enhancing the antiviral activity of immune cells. However, cytokine therapy can also have significant side effects, so careful monitoring is required. Another approach is the use of monoclonal antibodies to target specific immune cells or molecules. Monoclonal antibodies can be used to block the activity of immunosuppressive molecules, such as CTLA-4 and PD-1, thereby enhancing the activity of T cells. These checkpoint inhibitors have revolutionized cancer therapy and are now being explored for the treatment of chronic infections. Conversely, monoclonal antibodies can also be used to neutralize inflammatory cytokines, such as TNF-alpha and IL-6, to prevent cytokine storms and reduce tissue damage. This approach has been used to treat severe cases of COVID-19. Furthermore, adoptive cell therapy, which involves transferring immune cells from a donor to a recipient, is being explored for the treatment of certain infections. For example, T cells that are specific for a particular virus can be isolated from a donor and infused into a recipient to help clear the infection. This approach has shown promise in treating cytomegalovirus (CMV) infections in immunocompromised patients. Vaccine development represents a crucial immunomodulatory approach for preventing infectious diseases. Vaccines can elicit both humoral and cellular immunity, providing long-lasting protection against infection. Novel vaccine technologies, such as mRNA vaccines and viral vector vaccines, have shown remarkable success in combating the COVID-19 pandemic and are being explored for other infectious diseases. The successful development and implementation of these therapeutic intervention avenues require a multidisciplinary approach, bringing together expertise in virology, bacteriology, immunology, pharmacology, and clinical medicine.

7.1 Antiviral Drug Design

Developing antiviral drugs is a multifaceted challenge, requiring a deep understanding of viral replication cycles and host-virus interactions. The goal is to identify viral targets that are essential for viral survival but distinct from host cell functions, thereby minimizing toxicity. This chapter will guide you through the fundamental principles of antiviral drug design, showcasing the processes involved and highlighting key considerations for success. The first step involves selecting an appropriate viral target. This is often the most critical decision, as it dictates the entire direction of the drug development process. Ideal targets are viral proteins or enzymes that play a crucial role in the viral life cycle, such as viral polymerases, proteases, or entry receptors. Selectivity is paramount; the target should be unique to the virus or sufficiently different from any host cell counterpart to avoid off-target effects. For instance, the HIV protease is a viral enzyme essential for processing viral proteins into their functional forms. Inhibiting this protease effectively blocks viral maturation and prevents the production of infectious virions. Another promising target is the viral polymerase, responsible for replicating the viral genome. Drugs like acyclovir, used to treat herpes simplex virus infections, work by inhibiting the viral DNA polymerase. Careful consideration must also be given to the genetic variability of the virus. If the target is prone to mutation, the drug may quickly become ineffective due to the emergence of drug-resistant strains. Highly conserved regions of the viral genome are generally preferred as drug targets, as they are less likely to undergo mutation.

After target selection, the next step is to identify lead compounds. These are molecules that show promising antiviral activity in initial screening assays. Lead compounds can be identified through various methods, including high-throughput screening, structure-based drug design, and fragment-based drug discovery. High-throughput screening involves testing a large library of chemical compounds against the selected viral target. This approach can identify novel lead compounds with potent antiviral activity, but it often requires significant resources and optimization. Structure-based drug design utilizes the three-dimensional structure of the viral target to guide the design of drugs that bind specifically to the active site. This approach requires detailed structural information about the target protein, which can be obtained through X-ray crystallography or cryo-electron microscopy. Fragment-based drug discovery involves identifying small chemical fragments that bind weakly to the viral target. These fragments are then linked together or optimized to create a more potent and selective drug.

Once a lead compound has been identified, the next step is to optimize its properties to improve its antiviral activity, selectivity, and pharmacokinetic profile. This involves modifying the chemical structure of the lead compound to enhance its binding affinity to the viral target, reduce its toxicity, and improve its absorption, distribution, metabolism, and excretion (ADME) properties. Medicinal chemists play a crucial role in this process, using their knowledge of chemical structure and biological activity to design and synthesize new analogs of the lead compound. The optimization process often involves iterative cycles of synthesis, testing, and analysis. Each new analog is tested for its antiviral activity, selectivity, and toxicity. The results are then used to guide the design of the next generation of analogs. This process continues until a compound with optimal properties is identified.

Preclinical testing is a critical step in the antiviral drug development process. It involves evaluating the drug's safety and efficacy in laboratory animals. Preclinical studies typically include in vitro studies, which assess the drug's antiviral activity in cell culture, and in vivo studies, which evaluate the drug's efficacy in animal models of viral infection. In vitro studies are used to determine the drug's mechanism of action, its potency against different viral strains, and its potential for developing resistance. In vivo studies are used to assess the drug's ability to reduce viral load, alleviate symptoms, and prevent mortality in infected animals. Preclinical studies also evaluate the drug's toxicity and pharmacokinetic properties in animals. These studies provide important information about the drug's safety profile and its potential for causing adverse effects in humans.

Clinical trials are conducted to evaluate the safety and efficacy of the antiviral drug in humans. Clinical trials are typically divided into three phases. Phase 1 trials are small-scale studies that focus on evaluating the drug's safety and tolerability in healthy volunteers. Phase 2 trials are larger studies that evaluate the drug's efficacy in patients with the target viral infection. These trials also provide additional information about the drug's safety profile. Phase 3 trials are large-scale, randomized, controlled trials that compare the drug to existing treatments or a placebo. These trials are designed to provide definitive evidence of the drug's efficacy and safety. If the clinical trials are successful, the drug can be approved by regulatory agencies, such as the Food and Drug Administration (FDA) in the United States, for use in patients. The entire process, from target selection to regulatory approval, can take many years and cost hundreds of millions of dollars. The development of antiviral drugs is a continuous process. Even after a drug has been approved for use, ongoing research is needed to monitor its effectiveness, identify potential resistance mechanisms, and develop new drugs to combat emerging viral threats. Understanding the principles of antiviral drug design is essential for developing new and effective therapies to combat viral infections. By targeting essential viral processes and optimizing drug properties, researchers can create drugs that save lives and improve the health of millions of people around the world. It's also important to remember that the success of an antiviral drug also depends on factors such as the patient's immune status and the timing of treatment.

7.2 Antibacterial Strategies Emerge

The fight against bacterial infections has evolved dramatically, moving from the early days of serendipitous discoveries to a more targeted and nuanced approach. The rise of antibiotic resistance has made it imperative to explore novel strategies that go beyond traditional antibiotic mechanisms. We need to think outside the box, because the old box is compromised.

One promising avenue involves targeting bacterial virulence factors rather than bacterial growth directly. This approach, often referred to as anti-virulence therapy, aims to disarm bacteria, preventing them from causing disease without necessarily killing them. The rationale is that by not imposing direct selective pressure on bacterial growth, the development of resistance may be slowed down. Several virulence factors have emerged as potential targets. For example, bacterial adhesion is crucial for initiating infection. Interfering with the adhesion process, using molecules that block bacterial attachment to host cells, could prevent colonization and subsequent infection. Toxin production is another attractive target. Some bacteria secrete potent toxins that damage host tissues and contribute to disease severity. Inhibiting toxin production or neutralizing toxins with specific antibodies could significantly reduce the impact of infection. Quorum sensing, a communication system that bacteria use to coordinate their behavior, is also a potential target. Disrupting quorum sensing can interfere with biofilm formation, toxin production, and other virulence-related activities. The beauty of anti-virulence strategies is that they offer the potential to reduce the selective pressure driving resistance, while still mitigating the harm caused by bacterial infections.

Another exciting area of research focuses on harnessing the power of the host immune system to combat bacterial infections. Immunomodulatory therapies aim to enhance the host's natural defenses, enabling them to clear the infection more effectively. This can involve stimulating the innate immune system, for example, by activating pattern recognition receptors (PRRs) that recognize bacterial components. Toll-like receptors (TLRs) are a well-studied family of PRRs that play a crucial role in initiating immune responses to bacteria. Agonists of TLRs can boost the production of cytokines and chemokines, recruiting immune cells to the site of infection and enhancing their activity. Another approach is to enhance the adaptive immune response. Vaccines, of course, remain a cornerstone of preventive medicine, but they can also be used therapeutically to boost immunity in individuals already infected. Adoptive cell therapy, where immune cells are collected from a patient, expanded in vitro, and then infused back into the patient, is another promising strategy. This approach can be particularly effective in patients with weakened immune systems. The key to successful immunomodulatory therapy is to strike a balance between enhancing immunity and avoiding excessive inflammation, which can damage host tissues.

Phage therapy, the use of bacteriophages (viruses that infect bacteria) to treat bacterial infections, has re-emerged as a promising alternative to traditional antibiotics. Phages are highly specific for their bacterial hosts, meaning they can target specific bacteria without harming the host's microbiome. This is a significant advantage over broad-spectrum antibiotics, which can disrupt the delicate balance of the gut microbiota and lead to secondary infections. Phage therapy has been used successfully to treat a variety of bacterial infections, including those caused by antibiotic-resistant bacteria. However, there are also challenges associated with phage therapy. Phages can evolve resistance to bacteria, and bacteria can evolve resistance to phages. Therefore, it is important to carefully select phages that are effective against the target bacteria and to monitor the development of resistance. One approach to overcome this challenge is to use phage cocktails, which are mixtures of different phages that target the same bacteria but use different mechanisms of action. Another approach is to genetically engineer phages to enhance their effectiveness or to prevent the development of resistance. Despite these challenges, phage therapy holds great promise as a novel antibacterial strategy. The microbiome itself is increasingly recognized as a key player in defending against bacterial infections. The diverse community of microorganisms that reside in our bodies, particularly in the gut, can compete with pathogenic bacteria for nutrients and colonization sites. They can also produce antimicrobial substances that inhibit bacterial growth. Dysbiosis, or an imbalance in the microbiome, can increase susceptibility to bacterial infections. Therefore, restoring a healthy microbiome can be an effective strategy for preventing and treating bacterial infections. This can be achieved through dietary changes, such as increasing fiber intake to promote the growth of beneficial bacteria. Probiotics, which are live microorganisms intended to benefit the host, can also be used to restore the microbiome. Fecal microbiota transplantation (FMT), where fecal material from a healthy donor is transplanted into a recipient, is a more drastic approach that has shown remarkable success in treating recurrent Clostridium difficile infections. The microbiome is a complex ecosystem, and much remains to be learned about the interactions between different microorganisms and the host. However, it is clear that the microbiome plays a crucial role in defending against bacterial infections, and that manipulating the microbiome can be a powerful therapeutic tool.

Looking to the future, the development of new antibacterial strategies will require a multidisciplinary approach, combining insights from microbiology, immunology, pharmacology, and engineering. We need to continue to explore novel targets, develop new technologies, and harness the power of the host immune system and the microbiome. The fight against bacterial infections is an ongoing battle, but with creativity and innovation, we can stay one step ahead of the bacteria.

7.3 Immunomodulatory Approaches

Immunomodulatory Approaches

The fight against emerging infectious diseases isn't just about directly attacking the invading pathogen; sometimes, the most effective strategy lies in fine-tuning the host's own immune system. This chapter will explore the multifaceted realm of immunomodulation, a therapeutic strategy that aims to restore balance by either boosting a weakened immune response or suppressing an overactive one, achieving optimal control over the infection while minimizing collateral damage to the host. This is particularly critical in situations where the host's immune response is either insufficient to clear the infection or, conversely, contributes significantly to the disease pathology through excessive inflammation.

One key area of immunomodulation focuses on amplifying the body's natural defenses. In cases where the immune system is struggling to mount an adequate response, interventions can be designed to stimulate specific immune cells or pathways. Cytokines, signaling molecules that regulate immune cell communication and function, are often employed for this purpose. For instance, interferon-gamma (IFN-) can enhance the activity of macrophages and natural killer (NK) cells, bolstering their ability to eliminate infected cells. However, the therapeutic use of cytokines requires careful consideration, as excessive cytokine production can lead to a potentially fatal "cytokine storm," characterized by uncontrolled inflammation and organ damage. Another approach involves the use of adjuvants, substances that enhance the immunogenicity of vaccines. Adjuvants can stimulate the innate immune system, leading to a stronger and more durable adaptive immune response against the target pathogen. This is particularly relevant for individuals with weakened immune systems or for vaccines targeting pathogens that elicit a weak immune response.

Conversely, some infectious diseases are characterized by an overzealous immune response that causes more harm than good. In these scenarios, immunomodulatory therapies aim to dampen inflammation and prevent tissue damage. Corticosteroids, potent anti-inflammatory drugs, are frequently used to suppress the immune system in such cases. They work by inhibiting the production of inflammatory cytokines and reducing the activity of immune cells. However, long-term use of corticosteroids can have significant side effects, including increased susceptibility to infections, bone loss, and metabolic disturbances. Another approach to suppressing excessive inflammation involves targeting specific inflammatory cytokines, such as TNF- or IL-1. Biologic drugs that neutralize these cytokines have proven effective in treating autoimmune diseases and are also being investigated for their potential use in managing infectious diseases characterized by cytokine storms. It's essential to appreciate that the timing and duration of immunosuppressive therapies are crucial, as suppressing the immune system too early or for too long can impair the body's ability to clear the infection.

The gut microbiome is increasingly recognized as a critical player in immune regulation. The complex community of microorganisms residing in our intestines influences the development and function of the immune system. Certain gut bacteria produce metabolites that can modulate immune responses, promoting tolerance or enhancing immunity. Probiotics, live microorganisms that confer a health benefit when administered, can be used to manipulate the gut microbiome and improve immune function. However, the effects of probiotics are highly strain-specific, and not all probiotics are effective for all individuals. Fecal microbiota transplantation (FMT), a procedure that involves transferring fecal matter from a healthy donor to a recipient, is another approach to modifying the gut microbiome. FMT has shown promise in treating certain infectious diseases, such as recurrent Clostridioides difficile infection, and is being investigated for its potential use in managing other infections and immune disorders.

Furthermore, the development of targeted immunomodulatory therapies requires a deep understanding of the specific immune pathways that are dysregulated in each disease. For example, in some viral infections, the virus may directly interfere with the interferon signaling pathway, a critical component of the antiviral response. In such cases, therapeutic strategies aimed at restoring interferon signaling may be beneficial. Similarly, in some bacterial infections, the bacteria may trigger an excessive activation of the complement system, leading to tissue damage. In these scenarios, inhibitors of the complement cascade could be used to dampen inflammation. Personalized medicine, tailoring treatment strategies to the individual patient's immune profile, is becoming increasingly important in immunomodulation. By identifying specific biomarkers that predict response to therapy, clinicians can optimize treatment outcomes and minimize adverse effects.

Another promising area of research involves the use of cell-based therapies to modulate the immune system. Mesenchymal stem cells (MSCs), multipotent cells that can differentiate into various cell types, have immunomodulatory properties and can suppress inflammation. MSCs can be administered intravenously to patients with severe infections to reduce inflammation and promote tissue repair. Chimeric antigen receptor (CAR) T-cell therapy, a type of immunotherapy that involves genetically modifying T cells to target specific cancer cells, is also being explored for its potential use in treating infectious diseases. CAR T-cells can be engineered to target virus-infected cells, providing a highly targeted and effective way to eliminate the infection. These cellular therapies are highly complex, expensive, and carry potential risks, but they hold great promise for treating severe and refractory infections.

As we continue to grapple with emerging infectious diseases, immunomodulatory approaches will play an increasingly important role in our therapeutic arsenal. By understanding the complex interplay between the host immune system and the invading pathogen, we can develop targeted strategies to restore immune balance and improve patient outcomes. The key to successful immunomodulation lies in careful patient selection, precise targeting of dysregulated immune pathways, and vigilant monitoring for adverse effects. Further research is needed to identify novel immunomodulatory targets and to develop more effective and safer therapies.

www.ingramcontent.com/pod-product-compliance
Lightning Source LLC
LaVergne TN
LVHW022226200926
848481LV00006B/2139
* 9 7 9 8 3 3 0 3 7 9 7 4 3 *